Changing Ideas in
Health Care

Changing Ideas in Health Care

Edited by

David Seedhouse
*Departments of Community Health and General Practice,
University of Liverpool, UK*

and

Alan Cribb
*Centre for Social Ethics and Policy,
University of Manchester, UK*

JOHN WILEY & SONS
Chichester · New York · Brisbane · Toronto · Singapore

Library of Congress Cataloging in Publication Data:

Changing ideas in health care/edited by David Seedhouse and Alan Cribb.
   p.   cm.
  Includes bibliographies and index.
  ISBN 0 471 92068 1
  1. Medical care—Great Britain. I. Seedhouse, David. II. Cribb, Alan. III. Series.
[DNLM: 1. Community Health Services—trends—Great Britain.
2. Delivery of Health Care—trends—Great Britain. 3. Economics, Medical—trends—Great
  Britain. W 84 FA1 C4]
RA485.C445 1989
362.1′0941—dc19
DNLM/DLC
  for Library of Congress
                                       89-5362
                                         CIP

British Library Cataloguing in Publication Data:

Changing ideas in health care.
  1. Great Britain. Health services
  I. Seedhouse, David II. Cribb, Alan
  362.1′0941

  ISBN 0 471 92068 1

Printed and bound in Great Britain.

For Annmarie

Contents

List of Contributors

JOHN ASHTON   *Senior Lecturer in Community Health*
University of Liverpool
UK

TONY CADMAN   *Community Health Service*
Manchester
UK

JOHN CATFORD   *Director*
Heartbeat Wales
Cardiff
UK

SALLY CAWLEY   *Women's Health Team*
Newton Heath
Manchester
UK

JEAN CLEARY   *Institute of Health Care Studies*
University College of Swansea
UK

ANNE EARDLEY   *Department of Epidemiology and Social Oncology*
University of Manchester
UK

ELAINE FULLARD   *Oxford Prevention of Heart Attack and Stroke Project*
Oxford Centre for Prevention in Primary Care
Radcliffe Infirmary
Oxford
UK

ANN INMAN   *Women's Health Team*
Newton Heath
Manchester
UK

MICHAEL KEARNEY   *Consultant Physician*
St Christopher's Hospice
London
UK

ANGELA MARTIN   *Women's Health Team*
Newton Heath
Manchester
UK

DAVID METCALFE   *Department of General Practice*
University of Manchester
UK

JANE MORRIS   *Department of Epidemiology and Social Oncology*
University of Manchester
UK

PAM MUTTRAM   *Women's Health Team*
Newton Heath
Manchester
UK

KAREN NEWBIGGING   *Community Health Service*
Manchester
UK

P.G.F. NIXON   *Consultant Cardiologist*
Charing Cross Hospital
London
UK

RICHARD PARISH   *Head of Programmes*
Heartbeat Wales
Cardiff
UK

ALEX SCOTT-SAMUEL   *Consultant in Public Health*
Liverpool Health Authority
Liverpool
UK

BRENDA SPENCER   *Department of Epidemiology and Social Oncology*
University of Manchester
UK

BARBARA STILWELL *Department of Nursing*
King's College
London
UK

HELEN THOMAS *Department of Epidemiology and Social Oncology*
University of Manchester
UK

JUNE WESTLEY *Community Mental Health Service*
Manchester
UK

Preface

It is well known that health care is changing. Some changes have come about through developments in medical knowledge, others through reorganisation of the health care service, and yet others through a new emphasis on private care. Overall there is a steadily growing demand for health care, partly because of technical advance and partly because of increased life expectancy.

It is possible to identify two major trends in health care. One trend has arisen from the initiatives of carers working directly with people in need, the other has been generated from outside the health care system, by people whose priorities are not necessarily derived from the principles of health care. The first trend is a move away from a purely medical model towards a more egalitarian, more participative and broader conception of health. This approach is not only concerned with disease treatment and cure, but with ensuring that the whole process of care is as creative and enabling as possible. The second trend exists because external forces have sought to regulate the quantity of care available—seeking to limit spending. One consequence of this trend is that there are fewer resources available to many practitioners in health care.

Although it is not inevitable, these two trends often conflict, since economic restriction reduces the opportunity for improvements in practice. A potentially disastrous effect can be predicted if the second trend becomes dominant, and the priority of innovators in health care becomes financial cost-effectiveness, since this is bound to divert attention away from improvements in the *nature of care* itself.

The central message of this collection is this: to think meaningfully of efficiency in health care it is essential to consider every facet of care. For example, 'hospital output measures' take into account criteria such as 'length of stay' and 'material cost of treatment provided' in order to assess efficiency. But this calculation is simplistic and ignores other criteria which can also be understood in terms of efficiency. What happens to people during their stay in hospital (Do they feel informed or alienated? Are they respected as people or treated as objects? Are they educated and helped to adapt or merely given cursory information?) is at least as important as how quickly and cheaply they pass through the system. To assess 'hospital output measures', account must be taken of *all* the effects of care, not merely the traditional narrow indicators of success and failure. Without a thorough consideration of the goals of health care, and of how all resources—including human resources—are being utilised, it is impossible to make any worthwhile judgements about efficiency.

Many thoughtful innovations in health care are described in this book. They have been implemented by people working within the present health care system, and they form part of the trend toward holism, equality and autonomy for all.

Acknowledgements

It would not have been possible to produce this book without the help of the three secretaries who worked in the Department of General Practice at Liverpool University during the Autumn of 1987. We are indebted to Hilary 'Hils' Smith, Moira 'Moys' Currie, and Karen 'Kags' Black.

Introduction

What is this Book About?

The articles in this collection focus on changes that are part of a trend towards greater participation in health care. They raise two central questions:

1. How can these changes in health care be understood?
2. How can the trend be encouraged and further practical initiatives developed?

This introduction offers a response to the first question. The articles themselves provide practical examples and inspiration in partial answer to the second question.

If future health care practice is to develop effectively and have worthwhile goals, it is essential for carers to be sure about the standards they are aiming to achieve. In this collection a clear unifying picture emerges out of accounts of practical innovations in care. Each innovator justifies his or her initiative in different ways, using different terminology, but this book shows how each example of good practice has the same general rationale. The aim of the book is to bring into the open what most health workers already understand but rarely articulate—that there are shared central themes and principles which lie at the heart of all genuine work for health.

It is important to appreciate that although there are strong links between the articles there are also significant disagreements. This is inevitable in any complex living discipline. However, the common themes are greater and more pervasive than any differences in approach, or arguments about the merits of different types of treatment.

The book has been collated so as to cover as broad a spectrum of initiatives as possible. Aspects of self-help, health promotion, hospice care, nursing, medicine and community work have all been covered. The papers do not represent every discipline, which would be impossible in a collection of this size, but no discipline has been deliberately excluded. For example, the fact that more examples of clinical medicine are not included reflects only the pressure of space, and should not be taken to imply that the principles discussed are less important in technical or biological contexts—if anything the opposite is the case. It is regretted that a contribution from people working against racism was withdrawn.

The content of the papers is the responsibility of each author. The editors offer no critical analysis of the papers, concentrating instead on discussing the principles from which each initiative stems.

The Basis of Health Care

It can be argued that three themes form the heart of health care: holism, equality and autonomy. These themes can be subsumed beneath a key phrase: *valuing people*.

Holism, equality and autonomy are not watertight categories, nor is it suggested that a particular project can be only holistic, or only egalitarian, or only centred on autonomy. Most projects draw on each of these themes to different extents, and they also have aspects which are uniquely their own.

Valuing People

1. Holism

What is holism?   It is best to think of holism as an approach rather than as a distinct theory. Holism is often associated with the use of alternative therapies and contrasted with conventional medicine. This emphasis on the strange and unorthodox is inaccurate. A holistic approach can complement, enhance, and be a valid part of conventional health work: many practitioners working within the present health care system would be happy to be described as holists.

Holism is an approach which asserts that the best care can be given only by treating and seeking to understand 'whole persons'. Treating or understanding 'whole persons' requires a very broad focus. Firstly, it depends upon the recognition that individuals have both physical and mental aspects. Secondly, it depends upon some appreciation of the massive implications of this fact. Individuals are part of the physical world and in the midst of a complex set of physical interactions; but they are also part of the cultural world and in the midst of a complex set of historical, social and personal interactions. We are made of both matter and meanings and to complicate things further, we are subject to the material world and it is subject to us.

Sometimes it is necessary to limit our focus, but this should always be a conscious decision. It may be appropriate to treat some problems solely by clinical techniques, but this can never be all there is to health care. Those adopting the holistic approach also believe that people should not be cared for and treated without acknowledgement of the whole context in which they spend their lives.

The holistic approach has not developed independently from traditional medicine. Scientific medicine's success in explaining physiological and biochemical processes led to its dominance in health care. But scientific medicine has also been successful in showing that a purely biological approach is not sufficient. It has now become clear that cultural, behavioural and environmental factors have an influence on health and disease, and that there are causal relationships between the psychological and the physical. It is for this reason that holism must be regarded as a central theme of health care. It has always been so, even if this has not always been openly acknowledged, for in order to understand how to treat one part of a person's body it is essential to understand how other parts function, and in order to detect the causes of disease it is usually necessary to take account of a range of external factors.

The contemporary holistic approach seeks to examine and make use of new forms of health care, particularly those that involve prevention, self-help, peer group support and active partnership between the carers and those who are being cared for. It strives to examine psychosomatic factors in the causation and management of diseases and disorders, including heart disease and cancer. It attempts to locate all questions about health and ill-health in the wider contexts of lifestyle, culture and political debate.

The holistic approach is only one of three central themes of health care. It is complemented by the requirement to regard people as fundamentally equal and to consider the autonomy of unique individuals. A cursory understanding of holism might encourage the conclusion that the way to understand people is to see them only as minute cogs within a huge system of social, mental and physical interactions. We may be 'cogs', but it does not feel that way to us most of the time. We are also individuals who are responsible for our own actions, who understand things in particular ways, who give special meaning to those parts of life that are most important to us, and who make decisions and direct our own lives. This aspect, this feeling of separateness, of self, of being unique—which *all* people experience—must be acknowledged, respected and taken into full account if the most effective and moral health care is to be provided.

2. Equality

The principle that people are equal in certain basic respects is fundamental to health care. This principle is implicit in most conceptions of health care. Health care is directed towards meeting needs or fulfilling potential. It is not directed towards rewarding merit or serving special interest groups. Real work for health is thus blind to the many social differences around which human beings organize their lives. It is motivated solely by concerns which apply to all human beings equally. If the principle of equality is disregarded, if it is thought to be dispensable, then health care is debased. Discrimination on grounds other than clinical becomes inevitable, and what is worse it becomes acceptable. To decide to offer a treatment to one person rather than another because that person is younger, or whiter, or a man with a family, or not mentally ill, or not physically disabled, becomes justifiable according to the rationale of a 'health service' that has forgotten or abandoned the principle of equality. But no true health service can ignore this principle because equality is part of the core, part of the heart, of all true health care.

Unequal treatment, or discrimination, is sometimes a consequence of conscious decisions, but sometimes it is a result of unthinking habit or of bias built into institutions. A genuine concern for equality requires that the mechanisms by which these effects are produced be analysed so that all forms of discrimination can be eliminated wherever possible. A decision to offer a kidney to one patient instead of another might be sensible and justifiable on clinical grounds, but it is quite unacceptable, for example, that the least affluent members of society receive the worst level of care from the health service in general.

The key point is this: all people have biological potentials and almost all people are able, or will be able at some future time, to make choices. They have these potentials because they are human beings. People do not have equal potentials—a fit young man has greater biological potential and potential to make choices than an elderly man dying of cancer in a hospice—but all people are equal in the fact that they have some potential. It is absolutely central to the nature of health care that although some people may be far more productive, or far more kind, or far more able than other people, none the less every individual is equally valuable as a person. If a 'health service' moves away from this principle then it no longer has the right to be called a health service. It might be a business, it might be an industry, but it will not be a health service.

By emphasising the importance of valuing all people each article in this collection stands firmly on the principle of equality. Each contribution reinforces the idea that a true health service does not discriminate between people where this is avoidable, but opens its doors to all equally. Several authors indicate that their innovations are important precisely because they open the doors wider still, and extend further the range of services behind the doors.

3. Autonomy

It is often argued that a major goal of health care should be to create autonomy, and that if people are autonomous then this autonomy must be respected. In practice this might mean that if someone is suffering from a bacterial infection which means he or she can do no more than lie in bed, then a course of antibiotics should be provided not merely to clear up the infection, but also to enable that person to have more choices and to regain greater control over his or her life.

It would also usually mean that people, who understand the implications of what they are doing, should have the final say about the kind of treatment or care they undergo. Sometimes this general rule must be qualified because there can be conflicts of autonomy. For example, other people, including health care professionals who may wish not to be involved in certain procedures, must also have their autonomy respected. There is not the space to review these moral dilemmas here, simply to emphasize that in practice respect for autonomy means that a patient's wishes cannot be treated as a minor consideration but must be the starting point for all decisions.

To be autonomous means being able to direct one's own life. People are not entirely free to direct their own lives since so much of the world is beyond the control of individuals, but within the inevitable constraints of fortune, finance, culture and history it is a common human desire to be in as much control of one's own destiny as is possible.

The conditions for autonomy What are the basic conditions necessary for an individual to be autonomous, and how might a health service help provide these conditions?

For a person to be autonomous he or she requires three basic abilities, each of which depends upon both internal and external factors. To be autonomous it is necessary to be: (i) able to understand one's environment and circumstances; (ii) able to make (rational) choices; (iii) able to act on these choices.

All these abilities depend in part upon personal factors—for example a certain level of intelligence and perception is necessary—and in part upon factors of the wider world. For instance, a person who misperceives his personal circumstances (perhaps imagining himself to be far more—or less able—than he actually is) may be able to make choices (perhaps to pursue an unsuitable career) and may be able to act on them. But since he lacks insight and personal understanding will have a lower level of autonomy than he otherwise might. And someone serving a life sentence in prison might understand the environment, and might choose to leave it, but, as a prisoner, will not be able to act on that choice, and so will be constrained by external factors.

In order to have any of the three abilities a person must have been educated to some degree. Without education, without information, without explanations about what is happening around them no-one can begin to understand their environment. In order for people to be autonomous they must have a reasonable level of understanding of their situation, otherwise no rational choices will be possible.

There is no unanimous agreement about what rationality is but most writers in this field assent to the view that a rational choice is one in which an attainable goal is selected, and where the selection of this goal can be justified logically with reference to the prevailing external circumstances of the person. To have this ability a person needs to have adequate mental functioning, and also needs to be insulated from external pressures, such as stress, fear and depression, which might impair decision making.

In order to be able to act on their choices, in addition to education, mental functioning, and insulation from external pressures, people also need adequate physical functioning (or assistance with physical functioning) and their personal and social circumstances need to be such that they are in a position to act on their choices. If a penniless tramp and a person earning twice the average wage for workers in a country both choose to eat three square meals a day the working person has a higher degree of autonomy because he or she is in a position to act upon that choice. The conditions for autonomy are illustrated in Figure 1.

This brief analysis indicates ways in which the health service might expand its function if it seriously seeks to enable people equally to fulfil their biological and chosen potentials. All health workers are in a position where they can educate people, even if it is only about the reasons for and effects of the treatment that they are giving them. Health workers can seek to enable people to think more clearly, to conceive more realistically of the situations in which they find themselves, and can help them cope with stress, fear and depression. Health workers can do less about people's personal and social circumstances,

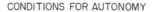

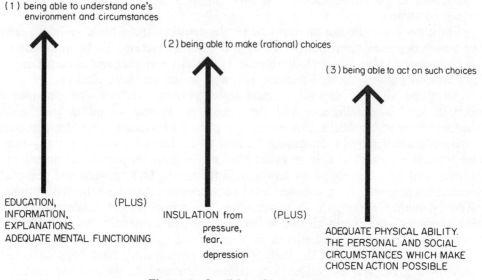

Figure 1   Conditions for autonomy.

although they might be able to advise them to pursue certain channels and courses of action of which they were previously unaware. They are also free to use their skills and their knowledge to campaign for social change if they believe this to be desirable. For example, many health workers are involved in campaigns to raise general awareness that the lower the social class to which a person belongs the more likely he or she is to suffer illness, to suffer more serious types of illness, and to die prematurely.

Every project described in this collection is concerned in a major way to improve the conditions of autonomy for the people it seeks to serve. In some chapters it is clear that increasing people's autonomy is actually seen as an important form of therapy for those burdened by disease or other problems of life. This emphasis on the creation of autonomy has to have a very wide focus since the conditions necessary for autonomy are very wide. Consequently, a health service that is explicitly inspired by autonomy as a central theme must have a different shape to a health service that is specifically concerned only to prevent disease and illness, and to lower the levels of morbidity and mortality. It is useful to represent the central themes simply, as shown in Figure 2.

Implications   The chapters in this book begin to show that health care might be significantly different to the way it is now. Although it is not possible to speak for the authors, there is a strong impression that the conception of health foremost in their minds is that true health is an ability to cope with and adjust positively to the problems that living generates. Most of the projects are dedicated to the reduction of illness and pain of all kinds. But in their common insistence that the key to genuine care is that people must be valued all the

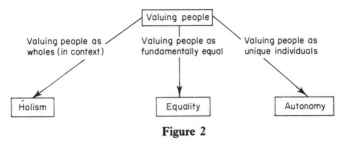

Figure 2

authors point to a system of health care that enables people to cope and to flourish, using the widest possible means to achieve this.

If it becomes generally recognised that these innovations genuinely reflect the heart of health care then the system must change. In part this change may come about as a natural evolution, but it must also be fought for by those who believe in its worth. This battle will take place mainly in the world of practice and not within the pages of books, but it will be inspired by theory and by the insight that work for health does have a common spirit and an immutable core.

There will be further problems of funding to be faced. The majority of the projects have had to engage in hard battles for money, and several face even more severe trials in the future. In addition, most authors write of the frustration they feel at being 'on the sidelines' or 'not mainstream' or 'marginalised', but this is the way of things when innovations appear. They can hardly expect to be accepted overnight. First they must prove themselves. This collection is a part of this process. Each article attempts to explain in different ways the efforts that have been made to evaluate the innovations. A range of techniques have been used. Few are as precise and exacting as the methods used by established medical science, but then the subject matter is very different. Finding ways in which to assess the impact of projects that aim to value people more is not an easy task. But significant progress is reported by several authors. And even if it is eventually shown to be impossible to create an accurate measure of this innovative care, it does not follow that valuing people is worthless, mistaken or wrong.

For the sake of coherence and clarity the book has been divided into three parts: Changing Medicine, Changing Communities and Changing Roles.

Part I

Changing Medicine

Changing Ideas in Health Care
Edited by D. Seedhouse and A. Cribb
© 1989 John Wiley & Sons Ltd

Introduction to Part I

'Treating the patient as a person' is a simple slogan with which almost everyone concerned with health care would wish to be identified. The four chapters that make up Part I of the book describe some of the ramifications of this slogan. We begin with patients and medicine, and with what is conventionally regarded as being at the core of health care: death, disease and doctors. The medical themes in Part I include chronic illnesses such as heart disease and cancer because these are representative of contemporary priorities, and because they most obviously require a change in thinking about the patient.

Michael Kearney and Peter Nixon write from a holistic medicine perspective on terminal care and cardiac care respectively. They demonstrate that holism is not simply a matter of employing different types of treatment. To see each patient as a whole in complex environments requires a change in objectives, in the range and content of explanations, in treatment strategies, and consequently in the evaluation of success. The extent of these changes is often reflected in use of language. The attempt to combine scientific and humanistic outlooks entails a certain amount of conceptual innovation, which is demonstrated at the most basic level by expressions like 'efficient loving care', which Kearney uses to describe hospice medicine. This seems paradoxical, since the concept of efficiency depends upon quantification whereas the concept of love is beyond quantification. Yet it is important to accept that in the practical world different outlooks and different sets of vocabulary often do make conficting demands in the same set of circumstances, prompting us to see things first one way and then another. It is only at the theoretical level that we can get away with viewing health care purely from an economic, or a medical, or a political perspective. Most of us like to make a virtue out of the relative simplicity and coherence of single perspectives. Holism means giving up this partial-sightedness even though it gives rise to complexity and conceptual difficulty.

Kearney cites symptom control and spiritual care as two of the essential elements of care, and he illustrates how these and the other elements of care can be integrated in practice. These two aspects of care are very different from one another and there is no simple way of balancing their competing demands. The former rests essentially on the medical management of the patient's physiology, the latter rests essentially on responding to the patient's concerns.

Kearney's chapter reminds us that in practice there is a strong link between pain relief and effective communcation and that these together underpin all aspects of care. He introduces the concept of 'total pain' to indicate the range of factors that cause distress, and that have to be confronted in order to enhance quality of life. Identifying this breadth of factors expands the possibility of creative care.

Nixon places the patient's subjectivity firmly at the centre of his chapter about heart disease and rehabilitation. Far from dismissing physical factors as irrelevant, he too seeks to locate them as part of a complex causal pattern that also includes emotional, lifestyle and social factors. At the explanatory level his work is genuinely holistic because he does not merely set out the diversity of these factors but he attempts to understand the interactions between them. In particular, he argues that the ability of patients to manage the effort they expend is usually underplayed in accounts of prevention and rehabilitation. He presents a broad model to explain the relationship between effort, excess arousal and physiological deterioration. Nixon makes it clear that adopting holistic theories necessitates a more imaginative attitude towards scientific rationality, and that there is a constant danger of our interests and explanations being dominated by those determinants that are most easily measured or quantified. Exaggerating the relative significance of the quantifiable is one of the most pervasive hazards of modern culture. It not only affects the way each of us comes to understand and appraise the world, but it is also built into the institutions which confer scientific respectability. In this way, social and political pressures exacerbate a common psychological tendency towards technicalisation and oversimplification. Nixon also demonstrates that it requires a tremendous breadth of vision to explore seriously the potential determinants of disease and rehabilitation. If we do not begin with the arbitrary limits drawn by what we can quantify, then we must be prepared to consider the potential importance even of those background factors that are not susceptible to the experimental method. Nixon's discussion of our cultural history, including the influence of the 'death of God', as part of environmental causation is an example of this kind of open-mindedness.

Each author treats the promotion of autonomy as an essential element of care. Kearney writes of the need, 'to increase, or at least not to decrease, the competence and independence of those being cared for'. In the case of the dying this value is an end in itself. In the case of cardiac or cancer patients it is also seen as an essential part of coping, adapting and rehabilitation. This challenges the conventional roles of patients and carers, and makes new demands on the relationships between them. To some extent these demands are met by teamwork on the part of the carers so that different facets of communication, moral support and practical support are shared between a group. But, by definition, promoting autonomy means that the teamwork should incorporate all parties including the patients and their families, as well as the professional carers.

The need to close the gap between professional and lay involvement in health care links together all the innovations discussed here. In Chapter 3, Anne Eardley discusses the role of cancer self-help groups in restoring patient autonomy, and in providing a valuable source of insight for the relevant professionals. In Chapter 4, Jean Cleary describes a Care-by-Parent scheme in which the attempt is made to share some of the responsibilities and skills of nursing staff in a children's unit with the chidren's parents.

Eardley and Cleary both begin with the problems of traditional hospital care; in particular, they describe how the environment, organisation and treatments of traditional hospitals can be perceived as threatening, can decrease rather than increase personal autonomy, and can thus cut patients and their families out. The alternatives are (i) to create a complementary non-threatening environment in which to foster patient autonomy, and or, (ii) to try to change the hospital environment by making it less threatening and alien. Eardley provides an account of one example of the former, and Cleary one example of the latter.

Eardley describes the complex psychological and social impact that the diagnosis and treatment of cancer can have upon patients. The threat posed to personal autonomy and quality of life are not met by conventional care, which centres on treating the disease. This discussion brings out very clearly the extent to which coping with disease is more than finding physical measures to tackle physical disorders. The very meaning of 'cancer' as a metaphor for all kinds of horrors poses a problem for the patient and others who are trying to grasp and to face whatever the reality may be. Yet there can be no coping without some process of coming to terms with, or making sense of, the experience of illness. The 'search for meaning' and emotional or spiritual support which Kearney identifies as vital elements of terminal care are an essential part of treating any condition which disrupts emotional equilibrium, whether or not it is actually life-threatening or physically serious.

Eardley demonstrates the intensity of the need for support and advice in her description of the telephone calls received by the self-help group. The people who phone do not know which way to turn, they may be exhausted, they are often deeply distressed and they frequently need practical advice about care or services. We are compelled to think that offering support to people in these circumstances should not be an optional extra, but as Eardley points out there is no inbuilt provision for either the support or education of cancer patients and their relatives. The forum created by a self-help group provides an opportunity for patients and relatives to share their ideas and concerns. The agenda is not exclusively determined by what is of medical significance, and therefore there is no artificial obstacle to the processes of 'making sense', of discussing the meaning and appropriateness of feelings, of seeking support and reassurance. As Nixon points out, these processes are not only intrinsically worthwhile, they are essential foundations for psychological and physical rehabilitation.

All too often the choice seems to be between being in hospital with no role, and being outside hospital with little or no support. This sharp divide reinforces the gap between professional and lay perspectives on ill-health. In the scheme that Cleary describes, an unusual attempt is made to narrow this gap; it not only seeks to develop the role of lay workers, but it also seeks to do this within hospitals by encouraging volunteer parents to take on procedures that are normally regarded as part of the professional nurses' role.

Cleary outlines the costs and benefits of the scheme and indicates that the latter greatly outweigh the former. There are disadvantages—some parents feel tied by the responsibility and their other commitments, possibly including other children, may be adversely affected. However, the fact that parents feel that there are considerable advantages of participation is strongly suggested by Cleary's findings that they would do the same again, that the experience raises their confidence in coping with illness, and above all that they feel they are involved and have a right to take part in, and know, what is going on.

It is particularly interesting that despite all these highly significant benefits, Cleary wishes to justify the Care-by-Parent scheme primarily in terms of it reducing levels of illness. Again and again we are all forced to see things through the traditional frameworks of medicine in order to influence or challenge those frameworks. Some of those who are simply opposed to the dominance of professional and medical values in health care will be wary of the scheme Cleary describes. They may see it as forcing medical and nursing priorities on parents and families. However, the reality is much more complex. The children, with the consent of their parents, have to undergo nursing care in any case. Some of the parents are volunteering, and being helped, to play a greater part in that care so as to complement their existing but limited role as companion and comforter. This scheme invites speculation about other ways in which families and lay carers may be able to participate more directly in existing health service provision.

The basic features of the chapters in this section are representative of the way medicine is slowly being forced to change. They are: first, the attempt to build a more equal partnership, and to close the communication gap between professional and lay carers; second, the emphasis on improving long-term coping skills, which means increasing rather than diminishing autonomy and which depends upon education; and finally, the widening of the agenda in order to understand (more fully) the complex causation of ill-health, and the complex needs of the unwell.

Changing Ideas in Health Care
Edited by D. Seedhouse and A. Cribb
© 1989 John Wiley & Sons Ltd

Chapter One
Hospice Medicine

MICHAEL KEARNEY
Consultant Physician
St Christopher's Hospice
London
UK

Introduction

'Hospice' is defined in the *Oxford English Dictionary* as 'A house of rest and entertainment for pilgrims, travellers and strangers . . . for the destitute and the sick', and so it was in medieval times. The word was revived at the turn of this century by the Irish Sisters of Charity when they began their work of caring for patients with terminal illness in Our Lady's Hospice in Dublin and St Joseph's Hospice in East London. The inspiring work of Dame Cicely Saunders and St Christopher's Hospice since the mid-1960s has established hospice medicine as an essential rather than a peripheral aspect of health care. This work heralded the 'hospice movement', a term which describes the huge increase in hospice-type services in the United Kingdom over the past twenty years.

In this chapter the essential components and different models of hospice medicine are discussed. These theoretical considerations are then illustrated in a detailed case history and commentary. The final section outlines the significance of hospice medicine.

The Hospice Concept

Areas of care

The 'hospice concept' describes a number of areas of care of terminally ill patients and their families, which may be listed as: symptom control, effective communication, family support (including bereavement care), spiritual care, staff support, teaching and research.

Symptom control   This is the cornerstone of good terminal care. Unless the patient's physical distress is expertly and effectively managed, the other aspects of care will be irrelevant.

Effective communication   Good communication is essential in this setting. This is evident in the context of the patient's relationship with the professionals caring for him or her but also applies in other settings e.g. patient/family, primary care team/hospice team. Good communication cannot be presumed and calls for particular skills and a positive approach.

Family support   The family, with the patient at its centre, is seen as the unit of care. Support for the family begins at the time of the first contact with the patient and continues after the patient has died in bereavement follow-up.

Spiritual care   An individual's spiritual distress is as much the concern of those practising hospice medicine as is their physical, emotional and social distress. Just as an individual's spiritual distress may be quite independent of any religious belief he or she may or may not hold, so spiritual care is not just the Chaplain's concern but a challenge to all the individuals who make up the multidisciplinary team.

Staff support   Individuals involved in hospice medicine need continuing support if they are to remain happy and effective in their work. This starts with careful selection of staff and continues in many possible different forms depending on individual needs and what facilities are available.

Teaching and research   The teaching of medical students, doctors, nurses, social workers and other health professionals is a priority of most hospice teams. Hospice units are especially suited for appropriate research into different aspects of this form of care. This is important if hospice medicine is to remain a respected and relevant aspect of general medical care.

Application of the hospice concept

Of the 140,000 or so patients who die of cancer each year in England and Wales, 60 per cent die in a hospital for the acutely ill, 30 per cent at home and only a small minority in hospices (Office of Population Censuses and Surveys, 1982). The terminal care of many more of these patients may, however, have involved one of a number of possible models that apply the hospice concept.

Domiciliary terminal care teams   These domiciliary teams may be linked with a hospice unit, work independently or be attached to a hospital. They usually consist of between two and six nurses with medical, social work and secretarial support. The team becomes involved at the request of the patient's GP and the vast majority of such teams then work alongside the primary care team in a consultative and supportive manner. The aim is not to take over patient care but to enhance the already established links with the primary care team in the sharing of expertise and advice while further complementing their role in offering additional support to that patient and family. Many teams offer a 24-hour, seven-days-a-week, on-call facility, which is greatly appreciated and rarely abused.

Most patients would like to die at home. Such domiciliary teams enable these patients to spend more of the terminal phase of their illness in their own homes and improve the quality of care in this setting (Parkes, 1985). In 1979 the influential Wilkes' Report (Wilkes, 1980) recommended that developments in hospice care should be mainly in terms of increased numbers of domiciliary terminal care teams, which are relatively less expensive to run. At that time there were 22 domiciliary care teams. At the time of writing, less than 10 years later, there are 170 such teams (Directory of Hospice Services in the UK and the Republic of Ireland, 1987).

Hospital support teams   The first of these teams in the United Kingdom was that started in St Thomas' Hospital, London in 1977 (Bates, Hoy, Clarke and Laird, 1981). In 1987 there were about 18 support teams (Directory of Hospice Services in the UK and the Republic of Ireland, 1987) and they represented an important step towards the dissemination of the principles of hospice medicine back into the acute general hospitals. The teams are multidisciplinary, usually consisting of between two and four nurses, a doctor, a social worker, a secretary and a chaplain. Support teams work in a consultative and complementary fashion. They not only affect patient care by advising on symptom control and offering support to patient and family, but are also in a key position to educate nursing and medical staff both informally on the wards and as part of the formal teaching programme. In practice, such teams find that much of their time is spent in 'supporting' the ward nurses and doctors themselves. Like domiciliary teams they are relatively inexpensive to run.

Continuing care units   These are wards or beds set aside in a general hospital for patients who are terminally ill. In 1987 there were approximately ten such units in the United Kingdom (Directory of Hospice Services in the UK and the Republic of Ireland, 1987). Their advantage, as their name implies, is that they allow for continuity of care for the patient who needs to remain in hospital. They also facilitate investigation or further palliative treatment (e.g. radiotherapy) if such is required. They are well situated for research and teaching but they lack the freedom to develop new initiatives because they are working within the same financial and bureaucratic constraints as the rest of the hospital.

Terminal care day units   While there are a few independent day units for patients with terminal disease, most day centres of this kind are attached to hospice units. By taking the patient for a number of days each week they relieve the family, offer the patients diversion and an opportunity to socialise, and allow close review and supervision of care.

Independent hospice units   In 1987 there were over 100 such units in the United Kingdom (Directory of Hospice Services in the UK and the Republic of Ireland, 1987) and these varied in size from six to 60 beds, from units that were fully NHS supported (approximately 20) to those that were completely independent, with the majority falling somewhere between either extreme. Hospices care primarily, though not exclusively for patients with terminal malignant diseases. Admission to such a unit may be on either medical (e.g. symptom control) or psychosocial grounds when it is felt that such care cannot be so effectively given in the home or in a local hospital setting. The admission may be for respite care with a view to subsequent discharge home or for terminal care. Hospice units combine experience and expertise of hospice medicine with a high nurse/patient ratio in a quiet, unhurried atmosphere. Most hospices have a home care team based in the hospice and working in the local community, an out-patient clinic and often offer day care facility as well. Such independent hospice units are, however, expensive to run and there is a risk of their becoming peripheral or isolated from main stream medicine.

Case History

The following case history of a patient whose terminal care involved a hospice service illustrates a number of points. These include the precise role and functioning of domiciliary terminal care teams and hospice units, the concept of 'total pain' and its management by a multi-disciplinary team, and what it actually means to 'improve the patient's quality of life' and 'support the family' before and during bereavement. These and other points arising from the case history will then be discussed in the commentary under the same headings.

Medical history

In September 1985 John, a 48-year-old married man who worked as a self-employed decorator, was diagnosed as having a locally advanced cancer of the bladder. After preliminary radiotherapy in January, he had an operation to remove his bladder, which was replaced by an artificial bladder fashioned from a segment of bowel. He made a good recovery after the operation and remained well for five months until he developed pain in his right buttock. A bone scan demonstrated that the tumour had spread to his right pelvic bones. A course of radiotherapy to this area in September 1986 in an attempt to control this now increasingly severe pain was ineffective, probably because the tumour had by then already spread more deeply into the pelvis. By early November the pain was incapacitating and John's GP prescribed slow release morphine (MST). Despite rapid escalation in the dose of morphine the pain remained uncontrolled. John's GP asked the St Christopher's Home Care Team to become involved. The dose of morphine was further increased and an anti-inflammatory drug, indomethacin, was added; this was soon discontinued as it caused gastro-intestinal upset. Further increases in morphine were only temporarily effective and by the beginning of January John was on a very large dose of morphine (MST 700 mg 12-hourly) and still in pain. As this situation was becoming intolerable for John and his family, hospice admission was discussed and arranged.

Hospice admission

John was admitted to a single room in the hospice on 2 January 1987. His symptoms were listed as his pain, which was described as severe, nausea and constipation. He spoke openly about his cancer and his realisation that it was terminal, and said that he, his wife and children discussed this. He showed little emotion throughout this initial interview and denied being either anxious or depressed by what was happening. He said that he did not have strong religious beliefs. When examined he was noted to be a co-operative, relatively fit looking man who was obviously in pain on moving his right leg. John's wife, Mavis, was present throughout this admission. She and John gave the admitting doctor and nurse details of family background and support and helped to outline John's family tree.

Assessment

The admitting doctor's assessment was of severe organic pain in a seemingly stoical man with a close family, which was not responding to treatment in the expected way. It was felt that combined medical, nursing and social work involvement was necessary in the assessment and treatment of this pain.

John's analgesia initially remained unchanged while the pain was being assessed and a baseline established. After a few days in the hospice John reported a marked improvement in his pain. He was noted to be quite mobile and to sleep well during the night. It was also remarked that what pain he did complain of occurred in anticipation of or during visits from friends or family.

During this first week John had a number of significant conversations with members of the nursing team. On one occasion he spoke of how he 'needed to be strong for his wife'. On another he spoke of the fact that his father had died when he was six years old, 'So that I know what it's like for the kids'. Perhaps most significant of all was a conversation he had with the ward social worker when he spoke of his memories as a young boy of his mother in uncontrolled pain. She had suffered from peptic ulceration and John vividly recalled standing in the kitchen at four years of age watching his mother roll around the floor in agony, and the feelings of horror and helplessness that this had caused.

A couple of days after John's admission it was his daughter Judy's ninth birthday and the family had a celebration on the ward. This was the only occasion during that first week that John complained of severe pain, which sadly brought the party to a premature end. On the following day Mavis, speaking with one of the ward nurses, described how difficult she was finding it to consider the possibility of a future without John. She spoke of how when she was nine years old her father had died of a heart attack in her arms while her mother telephoned for an ambulance, and of how in the months following this her family and, indeed, the world as she had known it, had 'just fallen apart'. Meeting John six years later when she was just fifteen and he was thirty-two had added further to her isolation from her family as they disapproved of her going out with a man 'old enough to be her father'.

Sadly, the improvement in John's pain was only temporary and it had returned to its original severity by the end of the first week on the ward. By this time it was clear that this was a complex pain whose aetiology involved psychological and social factors as well as the already known organic factors and whose treatment called for the skills of the full multi-disciplinary team.

Treatment and progress

9 January 1987   With the return of severe pain in his right buttock, radiating on occasions to his leg, John's slow release morphine (MST) was changed to 300 mg of morphine in solution every four hours and a tranquilliser (diazepam) was added at night. In addition, an anaesthetist from a nearby pain clinic was asked to advise on his pain control. The anaesthetists's opinion was that the procedure most likely to help was the insertion of an epidural catheter at the level of his lower lumbar spine through which diamorphine could be infused.

A couple of days later John, Mavis, Anna and Judy joined with the ward doctor, a nurse and the team social worker in a family meeting. This was presented as an opportunity for the children to meet some of the team caring for their father and for them to ask any questions they might have. Their questions ranged from what had caused the cancer, to why the pain was so severe and so difficult to control, to how the epidural catheter would work, to whether the cancer could be 'caught by hugging dad'. Mavis spoke of how she would very much like to care for John at home again if his pain improved.

Despite further increases in the dose of oral morphine, John continued to complain of severe pain. He decided to accept a trial of spinal diamorphine and was transferred to a nearby hospital on the 20 January. The epidural catheter was inserted and two days later John returned to St Christopher's. Over the next few days the dose was gradually titrated upwards until it reached 90 mg of diamorphine epidurally every 12 hours when he appeared much more comfortable and said his pain had greatly improved. Given the continuing success of spinal opiates, John was transferred back to the nearby hospital the following week, where a permanent, subdermal epidural catheter with an injectable reservoir was inserted. He returned to the hospice three days later. Over the next two weeks he and his wife were taught how to inject the epidural catheter themselves, which they managed without difficulty. Although he still complained of some pain, he said that this was 'not at all bad' and he expressed a wish to go home as soon as possible. During this time John agreed to meet and chat with a group of medical students who were visiting the hospice.

Given the continued improvement in pain, John went home for a day on 15 February as a trial run and this was successful. By the end of that week, John and Mavis were doing all the epidural 'top-ups' themselves and felt quite competent. Following liaison with his GP and district nurse John was discharged home on 23 February.

3 March 1987   The first week at home went well, with supervisory visits from the GP and district nurse and telephone contact from the hospice home care team. At this stage John developed a 'new' pain. This pain was in his rectum and came when he opened his bowels. An increase in epidural diamorphine to 120 mg every 12 hours made little difference. In addition, in discussion with a visiting hospice home care nurse and social worker, John acknowledged that his being tense worsened his pain and that situations which alleviated his anxiety, such as a visit by his GP, seemed to improve his pain. It was noted that there was an unwillingness on John's part to discuss certain aspects of his situation perhaps because they were emotionally too painful, and this was also felt to be exacerbating his physical pain. Following this visit, on advice from the hospice, John's GP started him on a regular tranquilliser, chlorpromazine 25 mg three times a day, in the hope of both helping the pain and facilitating communication.

10 March 1987   John was readmitted to the hospice. He was reviewed by the anaesthetist who performed a bilateral lumbar sypathetic nerve block for his rectal pain. An examination of the rectum performed under sedation showed that there was now a tumour in the rectum. Since John was completely free of pain he was discharged home again later that afternoon.

24 March 1987   Over the following two weeks the situation remained fairly stable, although by now John was generally much frailer. During one visit from the hospice home care nurse Mavis spoke openly in front of John of her fears of a future without him. He seemed aware of how she had been feeling and encouraged her to stay in contact with the hospice after 'he'd gone'. At this point he spoke of his looking forward to dying as a relief from the pain and struggle of his long illness, acknowledging that this must be difficult for his wife to hear. As the nurse left, Mavis asked her at the front door whether John would die 'rolling around in pain'. The nurse reassured her that he would not and encouraged her to telephone if she were at all worried about his pain. A couple of days later, Mavis telephoned to say that John's rectal pain had returned and that he had developed gross swelling of his right leg and genitalia. She was advised to increase his epidural diamorphine to 150 mg 12-hourly and that a hospice doctor would visit at home, with John's GP, in the next couple of days. The hospice doctor and GP, visited together the following day to find that the increased dose of epidural diamorphine had made little difference to the pain. At this stage John was quite weak and Mavis was administering the epidural 'top-ups'. He did not want to come into the hospice for a repeat nerve block so he was started on high dose steroids (dexamethasone 16 mg per day) in the hope of relieving the pressure symptoms from pelvic tumour. This proved successful and both the swelling and pain were much reduced within 48 hours. Over the following three weeks John's condition gradually deteriorated but he remained fairly comfortable. The district nurse visited daily and helped Mavis with John's nursing care. The children continued at school (which had been notified of their father's condition) but when at home and at weekends they also helped out and spent much time in the evenings lying on either side of him in his bed watching television. During this time there were a number of contacts by the primary care team and the hospice home care team but

Mavis continued to be the main care giver. John gradually became weaker and more drowsy and on the 16 April he became unconscious. The following day John died peacefully in Mavis's arms. Ann was present but Judy was across the road with a neighbour. The home care nurse visited by which time John's brother had also arrived. Mavis helped the nurse perform the last offices. By then Judy ahd returned home and she, Mavis and Anna spent some time with John's body saying their goodbyes.

Bereavement care

A week after the funeral the social worker known to Mavis made telephone contact and offered to meet and chat with her if she wished. She was happy with the offer and pleased to come to a first meeting in the hospice. At this she spoke of her sadness, of the funeral service and how the children had coped with this, and of her gratitude for the memories of such a peaceful final week in John's illness. She also spoke of her relief, saying that she could not continue to watch him in such a condition, when there was no pleasure left in life for him and recalled how he himself had said that he was ready to die. The social worker was able to praise Mavis for the care she had given to her husband during his difficult illness and her sensitivity and courage with the children through the time of death and the funeral. An offer was made of regular meetings of this kind over the coming months which Mavis accepted.

During the first five weeks after John's death Mavis found she had unexpected energy and in a spate of hyperactivity she redecorated their home from top to bottom. However, in her weekly meetings with the social worker she spoke of how difficult she was finding it to cope as John has always been 'the strong one'. She lost over two stone in weight and had frequent thoughts of suicide saying that quite a lot of her just wanted to join John, but agreed to a plan of coming into the hospice should these thoughts become particularly strong. With the passing weeks these thoughts began to lose their intensity. She had anxieties about Anna who was having trouble at school and Judy who had become very 'clingy', barely allowing Mavis out of her sight. Mavis complained that everybody was leaning on her and that she had not enough space of her own to grieve. During this time the social worker was in close and frequent contact with Mavis's GP and vicar, both of whom were seeing a lot of her, in an attempt to co-ordinate and support each of them in the help they offered in their different ways. Mavis's GP felt that she herself had become 'too involved' in the situation, 'more of a sister than a doctor' and needed permission and some encouragement to disengage. As time went by the meetings became fortnightly, occasionally they involved all three members of the family, at other times Mavis or the children on their own. By the end of June while Mavis was still acutely grieving, she had come to realise that it was not a matter of 'taking two days off to get over it' and to accept that it may take a year or more to find a new way of life. At this point the social worker passed Mavis's follow-up on to one of the hospice bereavement counsellors who would see Mavis on a continuing basis for as long as necessary.

Commentary

Medical history

Domiciliary terminal care teams become involved in a patient's care only at the request of the patient's GP even though the original idea of involving the team may have come from the patient's family or district nurse. The correct time to involve such a team in the care of a patient with malignant disease depends on a number of factors, including how advanced the illness is. In general it is appropriate to involve such a team when the aim of treatment has changed from 'cure', this no longer being possible, to 'care'. 'Care' in this context is a description of treatment (sometimes of highly sophisticated nature) which is appropriate to that particular individual at that point in the illness, the aim of which is to help the patient live as full a life as possible. The two main reasons for involving a home care team are for help with symptom control or to help by offering emotional support to the patient and/or the patient's family.

In John's case the referral was for both reasons, although primarily for help with his pain control. On average a GP will care for five or six patients with terminal cancer each year. While the primary care team will manage many of these patients without needing additional help, hospice home care teams may have an important place in helping with the management of the patient with more intractable symptoms or complex psychosocial problems. They also offer support to the primary care team in their front-line role.

Hospice admission

John's admission to the hospice was for assessment and treatment of his intractable pain and to give his wife and family a rest. Admission for symptom control and 'respite' care are two common reasons for patients coming into a hospice. This, coupled with hospice discharge rates of between 15 and 50 per cent of all admissions (St Christopher's Hospice Statistics, 1980–3), helps dispel the myth of hospice being 'the end of the road' and so allays anxiety at proposed hospice admission. In many cases, however, admission to the hospice either from another hospital or from home is for terminal care where home death is either not possible or not appropriate.

Hospices generally have a combination of single rooms and three or four bedded bays. Because it was felt that John and his family would benefit from the greater privacy of a single room, this was arranged. John and his wife were interviewed both together and individually by the admitting doctor and nurse. This modelled that John's family were part of the unit of care in the hospice context.

Assessment

While the admitting doctor had little doubt about there being an organic basis for John's pain, certain features suggested that other factors were also playing a part. John had needed rapidly escalating doses of morphine with only temporary relief of pain following each increase in dose. There was no clinical evidence of rapidly progressing disease to account for this. Nor, in practice, do patients with pain caused by organic disease rapidly develop tolerance to opiates given with sufficient frequency and regularity. It was therefore thought quite possible that pyschosocial factors were contributing to the pain. This hypothesis was made more rather than less likely by John's absence of emotion and denial of anxiety or fear when talking about his pain, family and his future.

The temporary improvement in John's pain following admission to the hospice, the apparent link between pain breakthrough and situations of stress, and the various conversations between John, Mavis and different members of staff each clarified further, by the end of the first week, why purely 'physical' treatment of the pain had to date been unsuccessful. This is a good example of a very important concept in hospice medicine, that of 'total pain' (Figure 1).

'Total pain' (Saunders and Baines, 1983) describes a situation rather than a symptom. The pain the patient complains of is understood as being just the tip of the iceberg of 'total pain'. Beneath the surface the different aspects (physical, psychological, social and spiritual, which vary in importance from individual to individual) fuel this pain. Unless these different contributing factors are recognised and managed appropriately the pain remains uncontrolled. The concept of 'total pain' and its management by the 'total' multidisciplinary team illustrates how hospice medicine attempts to integrate in its approach the polarities of either a purely medical model ('It's just about using drugs properly') or purely psychosocial model ('counselling, counselling and more counselling . . .').

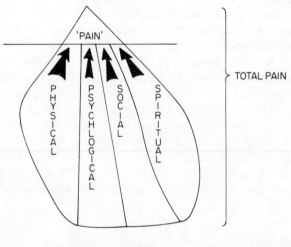

Figure 1 Total pain.

Treatment and progress

Treatment of the 'physical' aspects of John's pain necessitated the skilled use of appropriate medication and also, through the interventions of the anaesthetist, the use of relevant sophisticated procedures (epidural opiates, nerve blocks). This illustrates that the broadness of the hospice vision does not mean 'soft medicine' or 'the easy option'. Hospice medicine means, among other things, appropriate medical expertise.

The addition of a tranquilliser on a regular basis to help with the emotional aspects of John's pain does not mean that mental discomfort is an automatic indication to recommend drugs. By the later stages of his illness the links between John's pain and his spoken and unspoken anxieties and fears was clear. What was equally clear was that he could only discuss these anxieties to a limited degree. Psychotropic medication can be used in this situation, as with John, to contain and to lessen the intensity of this emotional pain, reducing its effect and perhaps facilitating verbal expression.

Meetings between the patient and his or her family and the ward team are often arranged during the patient's hospice stay. There may be one or a number of such meetings, which encourage communication and a build-up of trust and allow verbalisation of hitherto unexpressed anxieties. Frequently, as in the case of the meeting with John's family, it is the children who act as a mouthpiece for the adults in the group.

While John did not have a formal religious belief he did ask the question 'Why?': Why this pain? Why this time of waiting? These questions and others like them, like the pain itself, can be understood at different levels. Perhaps such questions indicate 'spiritual pain' and spiritual needs in the patient which must also be addressed. This is not a matter of easy answers or death-bed evangelism; rather, it means, whichever member of the team receives such a question, trying to help that individual patient to find for themselves some sense of reconciliation with their situation.

In addition, John's enthusiasm in participating in the teaching session with the medical students speaks not only of his generosity but also of how he as an individual needed to continue to search for meaning in even the most difficult circumstances. Perhaps this search was satisfied to a degree by the hope that others may learn from his experience, that 'some good may come of it after all'. Patients such as John are the inspiration of hospice based teaching and research whose goal, by disseminating relevant expertise and information, is the improvement of symptoms and situations such as his.

A risk in all areas of care and perhaps especially in terminal care is that the 'experts' will de-skill those being cared for, so undermining their competence and increasing their dependence. This obviously applies not only to patients and their families but also to other health professionals being advised by such experts. Any measure which increases the competence and independence of those being cared for is therefore of value. Policies of open visiting on hospice wards with encouragement to families to remain as actively involved in the patient's everyday care as they wish and the essentially advisory nature of hospice home care teams make good sense in this context. In John's case, he and his wife, in learning to inject his epidural catheter themselves, can be seen to have had the advantage of increasing both their sense of competence and independence.

The timing of John's discharge from the hospice, some seven weeks after admission, came at the time that he, Mavis and the ward team felt was appropriate. Central to this decision was John's statement that *he* felt his pain was reasonably controlled and that *he* wanted to go home. At this stage, and indeed throughout the rest of his illness, John's pain was never 'fully' controlled. However, to John his pain control was now 'good enough', which was a significant change to how it had been on admission. This was a result of the treatment and support he had received during his hospice stay but it also indicated an alteration in his attitude and expectations. Despite the fact that he still had some pain, and various other difficulties he experienced during his final eight weeks at home, it can be stated that his 'quality of life' was good during this time. To improve the patient's 'quality of life' in their final months and weeks is a central aim of the hospice medicine. But how can this phrase be more than a cliche and, more importantly, how can a patient's quality of life be realistically assessed? A model proposed by Calman (1984) has been found of practical benefit.

This suggests that the size of the 'gap' between a patient's actual experience and their hopes or expectations at any given moment (i.e. how it *is* and how they would *like it to be*) is an indication of their quality of life. The smaller the gap the better the quality of life and vice versa (Figure 2). In emphasising the importance of skilled intervention to relieve the patient's distress while simultaneously helping him or her towards an acceptance of the situation, this model affirms the main thrust of 'the hospice concept' while underlining the fact that it is patients themselves who judge quality of life.

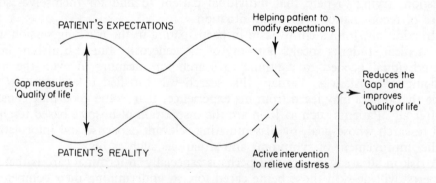

Figure 2   Quality of life.

Discharge home from a hospice, as in John's case, often involves a 'trial run' of an initial day or weekend at home as well as close liaison with the GP and primary care team. A lot of the anxiety encountered in both family and patient at the prospect of imminent discharge home arises from the difficult and sometimes frightening memories both may have of the final days at home before hospice admission. A successful day at home before formal discharge can do much to lessen such anxieties and increase the likelihood of the time at home being successful.

John's care in the final months of his life involved a primary care team, a hospice home care team, a hospice unit, a teaching hospital and a number of different professional disciplines and approaches. One of the functions of a hospice team involved in the care of a patient such as John is to share responsibility for the co-ordination of care at this stage. This is necessary as otherwise there may be a breakdown of communication between the various involved groups, leading to a breakdown in patient care.

Bereavement follow-up

It will be noticed on reading through John's history that in the earlier stages of his illness the priority is John's medical care. In the weeks approaching his death and obviously in bereavement, the emphasis changes to the emotional care of Mavis and the children. While both aspects of care are there throughout, this changing pattern of care is fairly typical. The care given to Mavis and the children from the time of first contact with the hospice was co-ordinated by the hospice social worker. In the later stages of John's illness this included notifying, with Mavis's permission, the children's schools of their father's condition, encouraging Mavis to articulate to the visiting nurses her particular fears about John's dying at home, and discussion about how to involve the children at the time of John's death and immediately afterwards.

Because of his previous contact, the hospice social worker himself offered and provided bereavement counselling to Mavis and her daughters in the weeks immediately following John's death, handing over at that point to one of the hospice's trained volunteer bereavement counsellors. This, as always, was with her GP's permission and again complemented the work of the GP and the vicar. Interestingly, Mavis's GP also needed support, albeit of a different kind, in her role at this stage.

Bereavement is seen as a necessary, if difficult, psychological task that each bereaved individual must undergo. Only a minority of individuals develop problems at this time and need specialist help in the form of bereavement counselling or therapy. Efforts are now made to identify such 'at risk' individuals prior to the patient's death in an attempt to anticipate and prevent the development of such bereavement problems by offering appropriate support at an earlier stage (Parkes, 1980).

Conclusion

The principles of hospice medicine outlined, illustrated and discussed in this chapter can be recognised as some of the most basic principles of the caring professions. Their re-emergence in the context of 'the hospice movement' has been described as an attempt to 'redress the balance of medicine' (Twycross, 1980). Hospice medicine aims to integrate medical expertise with effective support for the person who is dying and his or her family in what has been called 'efficient loving care'.

'Hospice' does not mean 'bricks and mortar' but a concept of care that can be applied in different ways in different settings. The aim of the hospice movement is not to monopolise care of the dying but to disseminate this concept of care back into the general medical services so effectively that it will eventually make itself redundant. This dissemination of the principles of hospice care occurs through the teaching role of hospice units, hospital support teams and home care teams; and it is hoped that because of this in the future not only patients with terminal malignant disease but also patients who are terminally ill with many other conditions will benefit from this type of care.

As a movement in health care in the United Kingdom perhaps its greatest significance lies in the fact that it is happening *within* the existing pattern of health care. The hospice movement is neither an alternative nor a complementary movement but an attempt to broaden the vision and scope of existing medical care from within.

References

Bates, T. D., Hoy, A. M., Clarke, D. G., and Laird, P. P. (1981) 'The St. Thomas' Hospital Terminal Care Support Team—A New Concept in Hospital Care', *Lancet* i, 1201–1203.

Calman, K. C. (1984) 'Quality of Life in Cancer Patients—An Hypothesis', *Journal of Medical Ethics*, **10**, 124–127.

Directory of Hospice Services in the U.K. and the Republic of Ireland (1987) provided by St Christopher's Hospice Information Service, Sydenham, London and sponsored by Cancer Relief Macmillan Fund.

Office of Population Censuses and Surveys (1982) *Mortality Statistics for 1980, England and Wales*, Series DH2 No. 7 HMSO, London.

Parkes, C. M. (1980) 'Bereavement Counselling—Does it Work?' *British Medical Journal*, **281**, 3–6.

Parkes, C. M. (1985) 'Terminal Care: Home, Hospital or Hospice?' *Lancet*, i, 155–157.

St Christopher's Hospice Statistics (1980–83) and Information Service, St. Christopher's Hospice, London.

Saunders, C. M., and Baines M. (1983) *Living with Dying—the Management of Terminal Disease*, pp. 12–13. Oxford University Press, Oxford.

Twycross, R. G. (1980) 'Hospice Care—Redressing the Balance in Medicine', *Journal of the Royal Society of Medicine*, **73**, 475–481.

Wilkes, E. (Chairman) (1980) National Terminal Care Policy—Report of the Working Party on Terminal Care'. *Journal of the Royal Society of General Practitioners*, **30**, 466–471.

Further Reading

Saunders, C. M. (1984) *The Management of Terminal Disease* (2nd edn). Edward Arnold, London.

Stedeford, A. (1984) *Facing Death—Patients, Families and Professionals*. Heinemann Medical Books, London.

Useful Information

Directory of Hospice Services in the UK and the Republic of Ireland (1987) St Christopher's Hospice Information Service, 51–59 Lawrie Park Road, Sydenham SE26 6DZ.

Care of the Dying—A Guide for Health Authorities (1987) King Edward's Hospital Fund for London and National Association of Health Authorities, 47 Edgbaston Park Road, Birmingham B15 2RS.

Changing Ideas in Health Care
Edited by D. Seedhouse and A. Cribb
© 1989 John Wiley & Sons Ltd

Chapter Two
Human Functions and the Heart

P. G. F. NIXON
Charing Cross Hospital
London
UK

> Coronary heart disease is not 'caused' by cholesterol or by hypertension as isolated variables. It is caused by a history of psychological and physical experience that leads to a breakdown of the entire organic system.
>
> (Allan Johnson, 1977)

> Just as the heart is part of a human body, so is the patient a part of a family and a society, and a person cannot be understood without reference to those others with whom he shares his life . . . social and psychological factors underlie all illness.
>
> (Annotation, *British Medical Journal*, 1971)

> The heart, overtasked by constant emotional influences, or excessive physical effort, and thus deprived of its appropriate rest, becomes prone to various alterations in its structures which necroscopic examinations daily reveal.
>
> (John Hilton, 1863)

Introduction

The contents of this chapter express the outcome of 30 years of personal effort. In 1956 the medical treatment of cardiovascular disorders was in the doldrums, and I thought it worthwhile to quit the conventional career of the standard physician-in-training in order to join Geoffrey Wooler at Leeds. He was determined to establish open-heart surgery, and the problems were formidable. In order to reduce mortality below a level of 80–100 per cent we had to find ways of pumping and filtering blood without destroying it; assessing acute blood volume changes within the patient; managing artificial respiration for days on end without tracheostomy; arresting the heart and getting it to beat again; recognising and countering the catastrophic effects of metabolic acidosis and alkalosis; dealing with heart block, arrhythmias and low cardiac output conditions; and developing the type of nursing care that is now the backbone of intensive-care and coronary-care units. At the same time, better diagnostic methods were needed and, in addition to the right heart catheterisation and angiography of the day, we learned to introduce needles into the left atrium, either through the bronchosocope, or by puncture of the atrial septum via the long saphenous vein at the groin. Indicator-dilution techniques were developed to detect shunts and provide information about leaking valves. Physical signs were studied intensively by graphic methods and related to the data obtained at cardiac catheterisation and open-exploration of the heart. We came to recognise an operable form of mitral incompetence from the presence of an opening snap at a time when the opening snap was thought to be diagnostic of stenosis, and many patients benefited. The hunt was on for the small proportion of patients with actual or threatened heart failure who might be rescued by the surgical correction of an anatomical defect.

Learning about homoeostasis

Hot blooded in the pursuit of technical excellence, we were energetic, righteous and arrogant. At the same time, we were intensely aware of two major determinants of success or defeat. These two determinants belonged to the patient and not to us. The first was the patient's will to live, and in the postoperative conditions of those days this could easily be exhausted by constant suffering and want of sleep and rest. The second was the ability of the patient's homoeostasis to go on defending the integrity of the internal milieu in the face of frequent, though generally well-meaning, assaults. The coping ability of the homoeostasis could also be exhausted by constant suffering and want of peace and rest. As Florence Nightingale put it, the patient might 'go off rather suddenly from some trifling ailment which just produced the sum of exhaustion necessary to produce death', and at autopsy we would rarely find an anatomical cause of failure to survive. The heart provides for effort, and we realised that demands for effort that were excessive and prolonged could destroy both the will and the means to live.

Forgetting about homoeostasis

In the mid 1960s the momentum of the advancing technology carried it into the coronary field, and a much larger proportion of the population—potentially the whole of an ageing population—became the subjects of investigation and treatment. At the same time the pharmaceutical industry broke out of its cage and convinced many of the medical profession that large numbers of ordinary people should take drugs for life to protect them from the cardiovascular consequences of prolonged and excessive effort. Opportunist dietitians jumped on the bandwagon and insisted that the main avenue to the heart was through the mouth and not through the mind. The relationship of the heart to effort was forgotten.

People who are exhausted by the effort of their lives, and driven beyond the limits of their homoeostasis and coronary competence, might be given anticoagulants, Atromid S, Inderal and a low-cholesterol diet, and never be taught to cope with the effort in the comforting ways that were a commonplace in former days.

A new direction: an interest in responses to cardiac catastrophes

I changed course. In the early 1960s I came to Charing Cross Hospital and became much less busy in the surgical field. I turned my attention to the problems of myocardial infarction. Still technically orientated, I set up a unit to deal with acute cases, and used it to define and establish treatment for hypovolaemic cardiogenic shock, but gradually it was the predicament of patients after cardiac infarction that came to dominate my attention. Like open-heart surgery a decade earlier it was unknown territory, and my commitment to it was the factor that put me on my present road. I started out with the common idea that angina pectoris, coronary insufficiency, myocardial infarction and sudden cardiac death were signs coming out of the blue, without warning, to announce the news that the coronary tree was rotten. The prediction of the next catastrophe was considered impossible, and life was seen to be fragile and precarious.

However, a period of observation soon made it clear that individuals varied enormously in their responses to a heart-attack. Some were failures because fear and family pressures compelled them to venture too little, while others defied these same influences and kept themselves ill with extravagent excesses of effort.

A few patients made an outstanding success of the illness, and ten years later seemed to be healthier and happier, physically more active, and more efficient in the business of living and making a living than they were before the breakdown. These gifted patients had little regard for the pharmacological fashions of the day: they did not regard themselves as pill-taking people. Their achievements seemed not to be related to the severity or duration of the cardiac breakdown, but to the intuitive ways with which their lives had been reorganised. They had made an audit of their behaviour and circumstances, and refused to go on exhausting themselves.

Rex Edwards' view

Edwards was one of the successful ones. He wrote:

> The heart attack did not come out of the blue, as these attacks are supposed to do: the ground was prepared by faulty living and the attack itself was in a way self-induced. This is not mere fancy—it is the result of much reading, enquiry, self-examination and analysis and careful deduction from known facts. I know for a certainty that I shall never have another heart attack, unless in some way it is brought about by me, either by allowing my physical condition to degenerate, my mind and body to become over-tired and overtaxed, or by permitting a too personal and subjective reaction to some situation of stress. This conviction has

relieved my mind of its most potent weapon for destruction: worry . . . Stage
two on my road back to health was the ability at last to learn to 'box clever'—
that is to deal with all stressful conditions, whatever their nature, intelligently
and constructively or else calmly to refuse to have anything to do with them.
This implies a degree of mental awareness and self-control which is difficult to
cultivate, but which, with perseverence, will always come. Instead of reacting to
a situation—one reacts with reason. In matters involving personalities one comes
to understand other people better, to see more of them as it were. Situations
which contain the seeds of hostility undergo a subtle and significant change: in
fact life itself takes on altogether more significance.

(Edwards, 1964)

The Start of Formal Rehabilitation

While I was studying these various responses, the late Harold Lewis of the
MRC was looking for a cardiologist to co-operate in the project of training
coronary patients to make the best of themselves, and he introduced me to
Alistair Murray, the Olympic coach and remedial gymnast. We worked together
and developed a practice of rehabilitation that seemed rational and prudent.
It was a great pleasure to learn subsequently that Lauder Brunton in the
nineteenth century, and Mackenzie and Lewis in the early twentieth century
had evolved or adopted the same methods. Nevertheless, the idea of training
patients, as opposed to treating them, and employing a gymnasium that was
not on a hospital site upset my colleagues, and the house governor politely
informed me that the project was to be closed to NHS patients. It took me
another 15 years to bring it back to them in the form of the now well-developed
occupational therapy service at the New Charing Cross Hospital.

Murray and I made a simple assessment of the patient's physical activity
and set about expanding it by training. The intensity of the training was
guided by the heart rate, and the exercises were not designed to carry the
patient above 60–70 per cent of his or her maximum capacity for effort.
Performing the exercises for half an hour three times a week was sufficient to
produce a satisfactory increase of the heart's capacity for effort, providing that
the patient was open to benefit.

It surprised us to find how greatly the heart's capacity for effort could be
increased after infarction, but it surprised us even more to find just how few
patients were open to benefit. In the majority, benefit was limited by factors
that we called tiredness and tension, and it was necessary to find ways of
dealing with these before the heart could take up its potential for recovery.
The prescription of exercise programmes became a routine matter, but learning
to understand the tiredness and tension, and enabling patients to break free
became for me the major objective of cardiac rehabilitation. Unfortunately,
there are no yardsticks by which these factors can be measured and made
legitimate in scientific circles. Furthermore, the reductionist attitudes of
scientific medicine and the limitations of the vocabulary used in a teaching
hospital were inadequate for the efficient exchange of information between the

rehabilitation team who are drawn from a variety of disciplines of conventional medicine and nursing, the auxiliary remedial professions, and complementary or alternative medicine. It was essential to create a map or guide to mark the position of the patient and the direction of his or her course at any particular moment, and the Human Function Curve proved to be a handy instrument (Nixon, 1976, 1982a, b, 1984, 1986a, b).

The Human Function Curve (HFC)

The Human Function Curve (see Figure 1) allows us to look at the patients and their problems and allocate each one to a station of health. They can be regarded as healthily tired, as exhausted, ill or verging (P) upon a catastrophic change or breakdown. The spectrum is shown as a curve related to performance and arousal (struggle, effort). On the up-slope performance increases with effort, but on the down-slope the arousal to effort causes deterioration. The curve is shown with a peaked top because most coronary patients can pinpoint the time or event that marked their 'going over the top' from healthy function into exhaustion and preinfarction ill-health. The 'intended' dotted line is drawn to emphasise the fact that coronary patients typically produce their own deterioration and breakdown by struggling ever more fiercely but always self-destructively to close the gap between what they can do (actual performance) and what they think they ought to be doing (intended performance).

This model enables us to recognise that some individuals have high curves and others low. A high curve permits great performance whereas a low curve invites exhaustion, ill-health and premature coronary breakdown. The handicaps that produce low coping curves in cardiac patients are commonly educational and psychosocial: migration; failure at school; poor mothering; poverty and struggle in childhood; loneliness; overwhelming coping burdens with lack of support, satisfaction and appreciation; and loss of prediction and control of life events.

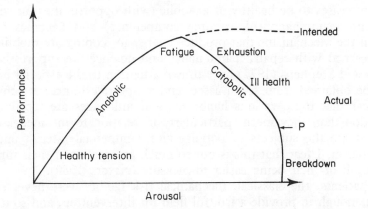

Figure 1   The Human Function Curve: a performance-arousal curve used as a model for a systems or biopsychosocial approach to clinical problems. P = point of instability where little extra arousal is required to produce breakdown.

The curve also enables us to picture the intrinsic and extrinsic drives that can get out of hand, produce morbid shifts to the right, and increase the risk of exhaustion, ill-health and coronary breakdown. The intrinsic drives include 'high levels of anger, anxiety, exhaustion and tension' (Nixon and Bethell, 1974); and the Type A problems of 'anger, anxiety, aggression, acceleration, haste, hostility, irritation and impatience' (Friedman and Rosenman, 1974). It is coming to be realised that these self-defeating human modes are common expressions of difficulty or failure of adapting and coping, and are not independent psychological entities.

The extrinsic causes of morbid shifts to the right that have been associated with excessive coronary mortality include blizzards; bereavement; financial hardship; and waves of unemployment. A high Life Change Score making us struggle to adapt more rapidly and efficiently than we are able is a well-recognised contributor to ill-health (Rahe and Ransom, 1978), and the harmful cardiovascular effects of information-input overloading have been described by Lipowski (1975). Karasek, Russell and Theorell (1982) have incriminated the aetiological importance of job demands exceeding control, and Ruberman, Weinblatt, Goldberg and Chaudhary (1984) the effects of high stress levels combined with social isolation. Eyer (1980) believes that the main causes of coronary heart disease are broad social forces, and 'primary among these forces are overwork and various kinds of social isolation'. Cassell (1976) described the dangers of exhaustion from excessive demands, particularly in those with inadequate social assets and a poor environmental fit. Weiss (1972) emphasised the importance of having the energy and information required for prediction, control, avoidance and escape. Engel (1974) showed how loss of control and prediction leads to exhaustion, with behaviour switching backwards and forwards between 'fruitless struggling' and 'giving up'. The fruitless struggling is associated with high arousal of the sympathetic–adrenal medullary system (S-AM) and the giving up (defeat, despair, helplessness and isolation) with high pituitary–adrenocortical (P-AC) arousal. Once the weight of the arousal outstrips the self-regulating, homoeostatic ability of the internal systems, the metabolism ceases to be healthy or anabolic (with opportunities for repair and renewal and maintenance of immune competence) and becomes catabolic, because all the mechanisms that produce energy for coping are mobilised, and those concerned with repair, maintenance and defence are suppressed (Table 1). Henry and Stephens (1977) have drawn attention to the especial protection that can be obtained from social assets and supportive human attachment.

It is clear that these various handicaps and influences are receiving much less attention than they merit, particularly in relation to the mechanical risk factors that are the subjects of popular and commercial interest and single-issue fanaticism. I fear that this is not so much an account of their importance but the result of their being easier to measure (Nixon, 1980).

In my patients, the classical, mechanical risk factors were never strong or numerous enough to provide a fruitful field for intervention, and so it was not surprising to read that they have a low predictive value and a role that cannot be causal (*British Medical Journal*, 1977). In my experience, relapses of angina pectoris or re-infarction were best seen as responses to psychological stress

Table 1 Catabolic and anabolic processes

Hormonal pattern during arousal

Catabolic hormones increase	*Anabolic hormones decrease*
Cortisol	Insulin
Epinephrine	Calcitonin
Glucagon	Testosterone
Growth hormone	Estrogen
Antidiuretic hormone	Prolactin
Renin	Luteinizing hormone
Angiotensin	Follicle stimulating hormone
Aldosterone	Gonadotropin releasing hormone (GnRH)
Erythropoietin	Prolactin releasing hormone (PRH)
Thyroxine	
Parathormone	
Melatonin	

Anabolic and catabolic states

Anabolic state
Increased synthesis of protein, fat, carbohydrate (growth, energy storage)
Decreased breakdown of protein, fat, carbohydrate (growth, energy storage)
Increased production of cells for immune system (white blood cells of thymus and bone marrow)
Increased bone repair and growth
Increase in sexual processes (cellular, hormonal, psychological)
Catabolic state (arousal)
Halt in synthesis of protein, fat carbohydrate
Increased breakdown of protein, fat, carbohydrate (energy mobilization)
Elevated blood levels of glucose, free fatty acids, low density lipoprotein, cholesterol (for energy)
Increased production of red blood cells and liver enzymes for energy
Decreased repair and replacement of bone
Decreased repair and replacement of cells with normally high turnover (gut, skin, etc.)
Decreased production of cells for immune system (thymus shrinks, circulating white cells decrease)

Decreased sexual processes
Increased blood pressure, cardiac output
Increased salt and water retention

Reproduced with permission from Sterling and Eyer (1981). ©Pergamon Journals Ltd.

(Myers and Dewar, 1975), biobehavioural problems (Lown, DeSilva, Reich and Murawski, 1980), and failure of coping with psychosocial burdens (Siegrist, 1980). Eating and drinking too much and smoking were seen as symptomatic of inability to cope with demands, and hypertension usually yielded to restoration of up-slope behaviour, i.e. to management that provided for the recovery of anabolic opportunities as did the stress-induced elevation of the blood lipids (Dimsdale and Herd, 1982).

Attempts to prevent heart disease by risk factor control have had disappointing results. The outcome appeared to be worse for the subjects than the controls in the MRFIT trial involving nearly 13,000 men (*Journal of the American*

Medical Association, 1982), and the *Daily Telegraph* reported (14 May 1983) that factory workers were at greater risk after heart advice in the United Kingdom Heart Disease Prevention Project. It is to be questioned whether the North Karelia Project reduced coronary mortality (Salonen, 1987), but it is clear that the Multifactoral Primary Prevention of Cardiovascular Diseases in Middle-aged Men did not (Miettinen *et al.*, 1985).

The importance of the psychosocial aspects is increasingly being recognised, and a lesser place given to cholesterol, smoking, blood pressure and the other mechanical factors (Kringlen, 1986; Siegrist, Dittman, Rittner and Weber 1982). This is just as well because these standard risk factors appear to have little or no relevance, for example, to the coronary problems suffered by Asian immigrants in London (McKeigue *et al.*, 1985).

Farrant and Russell (1986) studied some of the reasons for health information becoming unbalanced, and Mitchell (1984) examined the evidence underlying the extravagant claims for dietary prevention of coronary heart disease. He wrote

> When the salesmen call, in the guise of evangelists, you should therefore ask yourself 'Would I buy a second-hand vacuum cleaner from them?' I consider that you would say 'no', so I must end, as I began, with the words of H. L. Mencken: 'The most costly of all follies is to believe passionately in the palpably not-true'.

The understanding and acknowledgement of relationships between our external environment and the internal milieu invites us to share with our patients a systems or biopsychosocial (Engel, 1980, 1982) approach and to make much use of the processes of communication, information, education and support that are said to be inadequately developed in the biomedical service provided by conventional medicine.

The Biopsychosocial Approach in Practice

La fixité du milieu interne est la condition de la vie libre.

(Claude Bernard, 1867)

The biopsychosocial approach sees human beings as organisms living in an open system with their environment, acting, reacting and interacting with it day and night in a continuous exchange of energy and information. Energy and information are not uniformly distributed among human beings: supply and demand are variable, both on the part of the environment and the individual, and people vary in their ability to cope with the complexities of the rapidly evolving environmental systems in which they live. Some can perform or cope at much higher levels than others, and anyone can fall out of a competent performance trait into an exhausted or incompetent state. No one has unlimited performance or staying power.

The interactions with the environment cause arousal of the nervous system. The word arousal is used here to describe a behavioural continuum (Lader,

1975), extending from torpor, as at the left-hand extreme of the Human Function Curve (Figure 1), through healthy levels of vigilance and activation, into the morbid levels associated with exhaustion and illness, and reaching an extreme point (P) where the whole internal system, stretched far beyond the limits of healthy tolerance, is liable to breakdown as some small further increment of arousal carries it to snapping point (Nixon, 1982a, b).

The concept of arousal as a determinant of health and performance (ability to do what is to be done) is important. Hebb (1955) defined arousal as the organism's 'general drive state' and Kahnemann (1973) saw arousal as a 'reflection of what an individual is doing, and the effort he is investing plus what is happening to him and the stress to which he is exposed'. The relationships of arousal to performance have been studied or used in practice for many years.

I suggest that arousal-related exhaustion, illness and breakdown are widespread, and increasing in response to the turbulent changes taking place in our social environment, and the uncertainty they produce. If we fail to recognise these environmental threats we cannot develop a strategy for anticipation and prevention, and we shall have no alternative to the development of costly technology for reacting to established disease.

The Turbulence of the Environment

In her foreword to the study of the world before 1914, Barbara Tuchman (1980) wrote

> The period of this book was above all the culmination of a century of the most accelerated rate of change in man's record. Since the last explosion of a generalised belligerent will in the Napoleonic Wars, the industrial and scentific revolutions had transformed the world. Man had entered the Nineteenth century using his own and animal power, supplemented by that of wind and water, much as he had entered the Thirteenth, or, for that matter, the First. He entered the Twentieth with his capabilities in transportation, communication, production, manufacture and weaponary multiplied a thousandfold by the energy of machines. Industrial society gave men new powers and new scope, while at the same time building up new pressures in prosperity and poverty, in growth of population and crowding in cities, in antagonism of classes and groups, in separation from nature and from satisfaction in individual work. Science gave man new welfare and new horizons while it took away belief in God and certainty in a scheme of things he knew. By the time he left the Nineteenth century he had as much new unease as ease. Although fin de siècle usually connotes decadence, in fact society at the turn of the century was not so much decaying as bursting with new tensions and accumulated energies.
>
> (Tuchman, 1966)

The continuing acceleration of these changes into the post-industrial era has produced a social environment called turbulent by Trist because he was aware of the great increase in the size and complexity of our living systems, the growth of interdependence of its parts, and the constant awareness that sudden and unexpected changes in one part can destabilise the others. The result is quite a new order of uncertainty for both individuals and organisations, and an unprecedented challenge to their ability to cope with new levels of complexity, change and uncertainty (Sutherland, 1971). Koestler (1978) has described the striking disparity between the growth-curves of science and technology on the one hand and of ethical conduct on the other, between the powers of the human mind when applied to mastering the environment and when applied to maintaining the harmonious relationships within the family, the nation and the species at large.

> Roughly two and a half millennia ago, in the sixth century BC the Greeks embarked on the scientific adventure which eventually carried us to the moon; that surely is an impressive growth-curve. But the sixth century also saw the rise of Taoism, Confucianism and Buddhism—the twentieth century of Hitlerism, Stalinism and Maoism: there is no discernible growth curve . . . the most striking indication of the pathology of our species is the contrast between its unique technological achievements and its eqully unique incompetence in the conduct of its social affairs. We can control the motions of satellites orbiting distant planets, but cannot control the situation in Northern Ireland. Man can leave the earth and land on the moon, but he cannot cross from East to West Berlin. Prometheus reaches out for the stars with an insane grin on his face and a totem-symbol in his hand . . .

> . . . if I were asked to name the most important date in the history and pre-history of the human race, I would answer without hesitation, 6 August 1945. The reason is simple. From the dawn of consciousness until 6 August 1945, man had to live with the prospect of his own death as an INDIVIDUAL; since the day when the first atomic bomb outshone the sun over Hiroshima, mankind as a whole has had to live with the prospect of its extinction as a species.

> (Koestler, 1978)

René Dubos (1980) referred much to the relationship between rapidity of change and health in his *Man Adapting*. The essence of his message was that many people break down when they are compelled to live in a constantly changing environment and have to face an unforeseeable future in a new social context: sudden and profound changes in the way of life, whatever their nature, always reduce the resistance of the body and mind to almost any kind of insult. He observed that the health of primitive people depends upon the ability to reach and maintain some sort of equilibrium with the environment, and they fall prey to disease when ancestral conditions of existence suddenly breakdown. By 'a cruel irony of fate' in the heavily industrialised areas of the Western world, chronic degenerative diseases come to the forefront at the time when abundance replaces poverty: the chronic conditions Dubos had in mind were heart-attacks, hypertension, stroke illness, cancer, rheumatoid arthritis, multiple sclerosis, nephritis, leukaemia and mental disorder. Lord Taylor also supported the view that recent emergence from poverty was an important risk factor for coronary heart disease.

Ashley Montagu has highlighted the importance of crowding:

> the rate of change during the recent period of human history has greatly accelerated and immensely increased the problems with which people and societies are confronted. The first of them, upon which virtually all authorities agree, is the population problem. From the small hunter–gatherer populations of some twenty to thirty or so persons we have grown to populations in our cities running into millions. In these cities people in large numbers live in squalor, poverty and hopelessness. Disease, crime, violence, alienation are the usual products of such places where the disengagement of people from each other has become epidemic . . . the irresponsible multiplication of people has resulted in the debasement of the large part of humanity. The violence, the crime, and the corruption of our cities constitute but one evidence of a general breakdown of civilised humanity, evils which signal the loss of that humanity which once bound human beings together.
>
> (Montagu, 1976)

Dubos did not use the phrase population explosion but spoke of a population avalanche spreading over the earth, and pointed out how easy it was nowadays to suffer the frustration of our deep biological needs for territory and the maintenance of certain distances from our fellows. He felt that the evidence available in 1965 supported the hypothesis that the sudden increase in population density and the evolution of highly competitive habits might contribute to hardening of the arteries through indirect physiological and metabolic channels and promote cardiovascular disorders, heart-attacks and strokes. He felt that these vascular diseases were likewise encouraged by the pressure and anxiety resulting from social and professional competition, the effects of crowding and the complexities of modern living. He had more evidence at his fingertips than Halliday, whose work led him to link the growth of hypertensive and coronary disease to the progressive increase of insecurity and emotional tension due to altered conditions of upbringing in childhood and increasing uncertainty about job, income and status. It was becoming more difficult to resolve the feelings of insecurity and tension through progressive loss of satisfaction in work and the increasing neglect of biological rhythms. For him, the 'withdrawal of God' was far from unimportant in its practical, psychological and social effects. His thesis was that much disease and many incapacitating disorders had an epidemiology, but, unlike the infectious diseases, their causes could not be understood without taking the psychological effects of the environment into account. Henry and Stephens (1977) provided this review of Halliday's work and commented that his intuitive insights helped to inspire research that has now provided a more convincing accumulation of data. For example, John Cassel (1976) in his famous lecture on 'The contribution of the social environment to host resistance' has argued convincingly from the data that victims of tuberculosis, schizophrenia, alcoholism, accident-proneness and suicide have much in common: a marginal status in society. They have been deprived of meaningful social contact by a variety of reasons including high rates of residential and occupational mobility, broken homes or isolated living conditions, or by living in ethnic minorities rejected by the dominant majority in their neighbourhood. These factors have undermined their resistance. Widowers have a death rate three to five times higher than married men of the same age for every cause of death: it does seem that the loss of spouse increases morbidity from coronary heart disease, cancer, infectious diseases and peptic ulcer.

The alterations of upbringing in childhood mentioned by Halliday have been closely studied, for example, by Montague (1971) whose evidence suggests that being held and touched enough in infancy and childhood is fundamentally important for the growth of healthy behaviour. Being left alone in a crib to cry until the clock says it is time for a feed is not the best preparation for growing up, and the baby kept in close contact with the mother's body for long periods of time learns a great deal about her reactions to other people. Any breakdown of the bonding behaviour between infant and mother, which may occur when the latter is depressed, or shows rejection, can be as damaging to the infant's social adaptation as physical isolation, and the child who grows up without the experience of healthy bonding is unlikely to be able to pass it on to her daughter (Henry and Stephens, 1977).

Most people see work as the major area of life for satisfaction, and an interesting job is one of the most important of life's goals. Innumerable studies have been made of the different effects of dissatisfaction but from our point of view it is sufficient to see that they cause arousal, a rise of unpleasant tension that can exhaust the individual's coping ability and shift him or her from healthy to unhealthy territory as described in the section on the Human Function Curve. Kagan and Levi (1974) studied the reactions of various occupational groups to real-life situations at work and found that these situations could cause increases in the excretion of adrenaline and noradrenaline to levels that equalled those produced in certain tumours (phaeochromocytoma). In individuals, the level of adrenaline and noradrenaline excretion roughly paralleled the degree of emotional arousal. Beale and Nethercott (1986) examined workers in the two-year period between their learning that their jobs were insecure and actually losing their posts. They found a 150 per cent increase in consultations with the family doctor, a 70 per cent increase in the number of episodes of illness, a 160 per cent increase in the number of referrals to hospital out-patient departments and a 200 per cent increase in the number of attendances at out-patient departments. The older employees, with poor re-employment prospects, suffered more than younger and more adaptable employees. Of more specific interest to the cardiologist is the work of Karasek's team (1982) who showed that coronary heart disease and death rates were increased by jobs that combined high demands with little lattitude for decision making, and Ruberman's group (1984) who showed that the combination of high stress with low social support increased mortality after myocardial infarction.

The effect of disruption of biological rhythms had also been studied in many quarters, particularly in relation to the effects of jet-lag. Shift work increases the risk of ischaemic heart disease (Knutson, Akerstedt, Jonsson and Orth-Gomer 1986); and irregular hours induce bodily changes resembling those found in injury. If a sea-pilot is required to work irregular hours and maintain a high performance at unusual hours whilst still living in and interacting with the usual social and domestic pattern it is as if he or she is required quickly to shift across different time zones: the limits of adaptation are reached and disturbances of adrenaline, noradrenaline and cortisol occur because the body's systems of self-stabilisation or self-regulation (homoeostasis) are overpowered (Berger, 1987).

The loss of religion—the 'withdrawal of God'—may prove to be an important contribution to the epidemic of diseases of the heart and arteries. Every religion makes provision for the individual to withdraw into a condition of stillness, and to breathe calmly. The 'Prayer of the Heart', for example, bids us

> sit down alone and in silence. Lower your head, shut your eyes, breathe out gently, and imagine yourself looking into your own heart. As you breathe out say 'Lord Jesus Christ, have mercy on me'. Say it, moving your lips gently, or simply say it in your mind. Try to put all other thoughts aside. Be calm, be patient and repeat the process very frequently.

It is suggested nowadays that

> the cultural canon of our present society is heavily weighted towards upbuilding a powerful, rational empiric technology which involves the critical analytic information processor of the left hemisphere of the brain. Such thinking is quite necessary to achieve control of the social milieu and of the physical environments, but it is primarily cognitive, concerned with facts and figures. This left hemispheric way of using the brain is not well balanced. It may be the factor that enables man to increase his killing power without developing the balancing skills of communicating feelings and achieving peaceful rituals in place of aggression. Activities in religion and art, and imagination appear to involve the right hemisphere of the brain and give it a chance to offset the aggression and tension creation of the technocracy.
>
> (Henry and Stephens, 1977)

Another problem promoting arousal and a shift from healthy function to exhaustion, failure of coping and illness is uprooting. Durkheim's word 'anomie' describes a loss of desire to live in those who have become the 'disorganised dust of individuals' on the surface of the earth, through destruction of the genuine roots of social life in modern conditions of living.

> It occurs during dissolution of social order when the cultural canon has been fragmented and lost its authority. It is prevalent during civil war and violence and is associated with the breakdown of the family and disruption of attachment bonds. Lacking social support, individuals are exposed to excessive arousal of the fight–flight and depressive responses, and become vulnerable to mental illness and physical disease.
>
> (Henry and Stephens, 1977)

Lynch (1977), in *The Broken Heart: The Medical Consequences of Loneliness* has studied the increased rate of premature death from heart disease in the loneliness-prone; the widowed, divorced and separated, the old and the single young living alone, and children from broken homes. He has demonstrated that even the simple forms of human contact—such as a nurse holding a patient's hand—have proven effects on the heart. Lynch warns that in a society in which the divorce rate is rising and the family is fragmenting, in which social and community bonds are fleeting, and the children and the aged are neglected, our very physical survival is threatened. Truly, he concludes we must learn to live together, or we shall die, prematurely or alone. His opinions remind me of Montagu.

> The other reason for trying to understand our aggressiveness is that the time has come when we must. Finally after some five or six million years of human existence on this planet, human violence threatens to take the reins from human cooperativeness and inventiveness and drive us into extinction. Until now, we have balanced out fairly well as a species, and in fact we have continued to grow and develop. But now, with our human ingenuity working full blast, we have devised ways to wipe out ourselves with a speed and thoroughness unknown to us before. If we want this unpleasant planet to be inhabited by any of our descendants, we have no choice but to arrive at some better understanding of our natures. Or at least to keep on trying.
>
> (Montagu, 1976)

Migration is another potential cause of a marginal position in society, and an increased risk of coronary disease. For example, Asian immigrants to England and Wales have a high mortality from coronary heart disease, and this increase over the level of the British population is not caused by the larger proportion of non-smokers and vegetarians among them! (McKeigue *et al.*, 1985). A most useful and wide-ranging study of migration and its effects upon health are found in Zwingmann's (1977) *Uprooting and Related Phenomena*.

The medical services are not unaware of these various charges. The Royal College of General Practitioners has published a paper on the need for adaptation in medical practice whose introductory words are

> Society is changing probably faster than most people realise. There are demographic changes, morbidity changes, structural changes, educational changes, changes in attitudes to health, behavioural changes, politico-economic changes— and behind all these, subtle ecological changes. All have health service implications.
>
> (Metcalfe, 1981)

The Internal Milieu

The treadwheel (Figure 2) is a useful model for creating concepts of the processes involved in illness and rehabilitation. It can represent the burdens of arousal generated by the activities of living and making a living. The figure on the left is in control and in good health: he can take a vigorous part in the world around him and yet keep his internal milieu in the balanced, orderly stable and competent condition we call anabolic (see Table 1). His station is

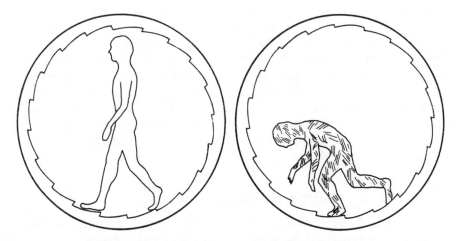

Figure 2   The treadwheel: a useful model for considering the requirements for a stable
and orderly internal milieu and an anabolic system (figure on left), and for
disorder with catabolic degradation of function (figure on right).

on the up-slope of the HFC. He may have a high curve and enjoy hardiness,
a resistance to illness linked with three particular qualities (Kobasa, Maddi
and Kahn, 1982): commitment, control and challenge. By 'commitment',
Kobasa means the disposition to become active in what is going on, rather
than withdrawn, and being unable to give up easily under pressure. 'Control'
is the tendency to feel and act as if one has influence rather than helplessness
in the varied contingencies of life. 'Challenge' is the disposition to believe that
change rather than stability is the normal way of life, and the possession of
sufficient energy to regard it as an interesting and rewarding incentive to
growth. If Kobasa is right, the anatomy of hardiness looks very much like the
anatomy of courage, and I imagine that the one is as vulnerable as the other
to exhaustion.

The figure on the left also enjoys, by good fortune or achievement, enough
satisfaction of his needs to live with a tolerably low level of arousal. From my
point of view, the commonest causes of arousal-related illness in cardiological
practice are failure of achievement and esteem from living without the ability
to develop talents and achieve a sense of worth.

His potential for survival also depends upon the three assets required for
the maintenance of health and freedom in a turbulent and uncertain society.
The first is autonomy, the privilege of choice and self-direction. The second
is self-organisation, the capacity for organising energy and information to adapt
and cope in such a way as to produce a favourable outcome. The third is a
strong homoeostatic system that can maintain the order and stability of the
internal milieu in challenging conditions of high and prolonged arousal.

The figure on the right of Figure 2 portrays the individual on the down-
slope of the HFC. His performance is falling, and the rate of the decline
accelerates with every surge of effort to raise it to the level he intends. His
talent for struggling is now undermining him and he does not know why. He

may put great energy into a project and use its success to reassure himself, but fails to see that the energy was drawn from ever-diminishing reserves.

The arousal rises with every fresh struggle (S-AM activation) and defeat (P-AC activation) and, unchecked, produces cascades of self-defeating and self-destructive changes, and vicious circles of degradation that affect every part of the human organism. Rehabilitation depends upon their recognition and management. Various aspects will be considered briefly under the headings of adaptation and habituation, behaviour and social relationships, emotions and the internal milieu, autonomy, hyperventilation, and destabilisation of the cardiovascular system.

Adaptation and Habituation

The organism reduces vigilance, the need for energy and the amount of information to be processed by adapting to change and habituating—reducing responsivity—to stimuli. In the state of exhaustion on the down-slope of the HFC these processes fail to modulate responses as they should and so the arousal flourishes: for example, becoming upset by a family member in a familiar way may now produce an escalation of anger with an unchecked rise of blood pressure and coagulability that can produce such a catastrophe as a stroke illness.

The observation of patients' blood pressure charts (Figure 3) suggests that the sleep loss of high arousal states is the key to the failure of adaptation and habituation. Its opening of the door to catabolic degradation is well known (Adam and Oswald, 1984), and its specific relationship to coronary heart disease is being unravelled (Freeman and Nixon, 1987a; Jenkins et al., 1983).

Exhaustion is often spotlighted in management and public life when deterioration of performance and failure of adaptation produce noticeable effects, but the cause is usually attributed to ageing, incompetence, alcohol or viral infection. Appels (1983) has studied its importance in the year before myocardial infarction, and Siegrist et al. (1982) have reported the social causes of the exhausting distress that has occurred in patients with early myocardial infarction.

Behaviour and Social Relationships

Lipowski's (1975) list of the effects of information-input overloading provides a useful basis of classification for cardiological work. The brain's information processing becomes less efficient, fewer problems are solved by our 'automatic pilots', and we become more easily aroused—hot and bothered—about more things. Thus the heart is given more work to do, and the product of heart rate and blood pressure becomes greater for a given amount of effort. These processes are called deconditioning.

Performance is impaired by loss of energy and stamina, loss of speed and accuracy of response, and increasing feelings of resentment and paranoia. Vigilance and restlessness increase. Discriminative powers deteriorate and the subject becomes less capable of managing time and resources efficiently.

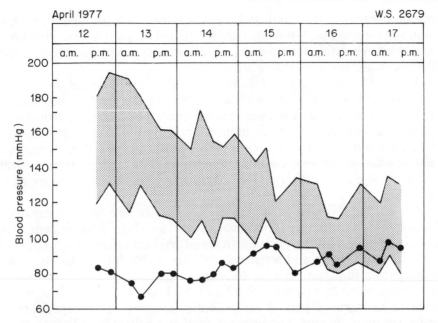

Figure 3 Businessman aged 54 years. The blood pressure (stippled area) and heart rate
(●—●) changes during a sleeping/resting regimen prescribed for recovery from
a period of homoeostasis violation induced by exhausting effort and loss of
sleep during a business tour in the Middle East. From 12 to 14 April the sleep
required hypnotics but from 15 to 17 April it occurred naturally. Afterwards
the blood pressure returned to its customary level of 110/60 and remained
there. Without a sleeping/resting regimen in such cases, the blood pressure
usually remains raised, becomes resistant to hypotensive drug therapy and
increases with further effort.

Judgement is impaired. The loss of leadership qualities compels more reliance
to be placed on rank and seniority. Reducing adaptability causes defences to
be erected against change, and a tendency to dwell in the past instead of in
the future. There is a temptation to sit around eating, drinking and talking
too much instead of getting on with the task in hand. Aggression flares up
and destroys the goodwill of potential allies. Maladaptive coping habits are
commonly adopted: they include acquiescence in sleep deprivation, denial of
major problems and indulgence in exhausting displacement activities. People
in this phase of exhaustion are prone to hurl themselves into ill-judged physical
effort, producing the risk of myocardial infarction and cardiac arrest. Total
failure of coping is very close when the patient feels desperately trapped,
unable to carry on and unable to opt out. Feeling trapped, he or she is likely
to hyperventilate, and the hyperventilation can trigger off coronary arterial
spasm and fatal arrhythmia.

Social disorganisation occurs when subjects stop listening to others. They
lose insight, become impossible to live with or work with, and neurotic traits
get out of hand.

Neurohumorally, S-AM and P-AC arousal can rise to extremely high, phaeochromocytoma-like levels of activity. It becomes extremely difficult for the body's self-regulating mechanisms (homoeostasis) to withstand the catabolic assaults and maintain a healthy internal milieu.

It is likely that the changes of behaviour and social relationships found on the down-slope of the HFC modify the function of the cerebral hemispheres, and suffer further degradation from this disorder. The feeling is growing that exhaustion and high arousal states induce limbic dysfunction with loss of left-hemispheric inhibition (Gruzelier *et al.*, 1986), and an increase of left sympathetic stimulation that encourages coronary vasoconstriction and malignant cardiac arrhythmia (Lane and Schwartz, 1987; Malliani, 1982; Verrier, Hagestad and Lown, 1987).

Patients on the down-slope of the HFC often appear to be incapable of recognising the relationships between events in their environment, their emotional responses and the psychological and physical effects they suffer. The word alexithymia (Henry and Stephens, 1977) probably fits this handicap best: it certainly is an important barrier to rehabilitation.

The Type A behaviour pattern (Friedman and Rosenman, 1974) is sometimes regarded as an intrinsic part of an individual's nature, an independent risk factor for coronary disease, but in rehabilitation I believe it is best treated as a manifestation of down-slope behaviour. Henry (1987) has also provided an up-to-date review of psychological factors and coronary heart disease.

Emotions and the Internal Milieu

I use the word arousal in rehabilitation because the patient on the down-slope of the HFC can slip in and out of fear, anxiety and anger on the one hand, or grief, humiliation, subordination, hurt or despair on the other, with amazing speed; sometimes denying emotional upset, or withdrawing from it by hyperventilating as did Dr Livingstone when his arm was mauled by a lion. The high level of the behavioural arousal, its variability and its instability are the keynotes. I have seen an able counsellor, an inpatient herself, report a complicated series of observations and make recommendations with startling clarity about a fellow patient: a few moments later she hyperventilated and became no more competent than an angrily upset and bewildered child when it came to a discussion of her own symptoms.

We owe Henry (1975, 1982, 1986) a great debt for unravelling the linkages between the emotions on the down-slope of the HFC, where the neuroendocrine responses are unlikely to be well governed, and illness. First of all, he showed that social interaction could produce states of high and sustained arousal to which the neuroendocrine system responded in ways that produced acute and chronic disturbances of cardiovascular function, including sudden death, and sustained hypertension with arteriosclerotic lesions in the heart. Later he developed the theme summarised here:

Psychosocial stimulation produces a number of neuroendocrine responses. The first is the pituitary–adrenocortical system (P-AC), which responds to situations that create a high degree of uncertainty and are linked with feelings of defeat, despair, loss and isolation. The second is the catecholamine fight–flight sympathetic–adrenal medullary system (S-AM): it is crucially involved in situations that require attention or vigilance. When the situation requires an aggressive, directed attack, then noradrenaline (alpha-adrenergic, vasoconstrictive) is the more important catecholamine. When uncertainty and anxiety are dominant, both adrenaline (beta-adrenergic, increasing heart contractility and rate) and noradrenaline are involved. The following concepts are useful:

1. Effort without distress is a happy state accompanied by catecholamine secretion. P-AC activity may be suppressed.
2. Effort with distress—the common product of daily hassles in our environmental system—is associated with increased S-AM and P-AC activity.
3. Distress without effort—giving up, feeling helpless and isolated, losing social rank and assets, playing dead—is accompanied by high P-AC activity and high levels of cortisol.

The third neuroendocrine system of practical interest is the psychoneuroimmune system. It appears that activation of the P-AC system is associated with immune incompetence (Freeman and Nixon, 1987b) and so it is not surprising that musculo-skeletal disorders and arthritis are found so commonly in coronary patients.

The fourth neuroendocrine system of importance in cardiac rehabilitation is the pituitary–gonadotrophic. The control of androgens, oestrogens and progesterone appear to be influenced by the security and sense of control that an individual perceives in his or her life situation. In men the achievement of security and control—the successful expression of autonomy—is associated with increased secretion of testosterone and the added rewards of greater stamina, concentration and sexual ability (Freeman and Nixon, 1987a).

Catabolic levels of arousal, where homoeostasic self-regulation is incompetent, must be seen as self-defeating, and, if ignored, self-destructive. The major changes are presented in Table 1. The cardiovascular consequences include: systolic and diastolic hypertension, increased tissue demands for oxygen, increased heart rate and stroke volume, and increased serum uric acid, cholesterol and free fatty acids, plasma glucose, platelet adhesiveness, and blood viscosity. Constriction of the peripheral resistance and the capacitance vessels of the body can occur. It is thought that this catabolic internal milieu damages the arteries and impairs left ventricular function. Eventually a point of instability is reached where a catastrophe can be initiated by a small increment of change favouring thrombosis and vasospasm. The *coup de grace* sometimes takes the form of a fatal arrhythmia or attack of coronary vasospasm induced by hyperventilation at a time of acute or chronic arousal when the homoeostatic defences are reduced (Nixon, 1982a, 1983b).

There are many contributions to this hypothesis, and important sources include Friedman and Rosenman (1974), Buell and Eliot (1980) and the publications by Raab (1969), Levi (1972), Kagan and Levi (1974), Groen (1976), Henry and Meehan (1981), Sterling and Eyer (1981), Karasek *et al.* (1982), Kagan (1982) and Dimsdale and Herd (1982).

It is little wonder that Osler regarded coronary artery disease as the nemesis through which nature extracts retribution for the violation of her laws.

Autonomy

The downward shift from health that deepens our exhaustion, makes us ill, damages tissues and ultimately takes away life, clearly destroys autonomy. Without autonomy and self-organisation we cannot take charge, mobilise our defences, and fight for the recovery of stable and orderly relationships with the external environment. A grave fault of technological cardiology is its failure to mobilise these resources. For example, admission to a coronary care unit has such a strong adverse influence that it subsequently makes little or no difference to outcome whether the diagnosis is 'myocardial infarction' or 'not infarction'. A year after coronary arteriography, it makes little difference to employment outcome whether the verdict is 'normal' or 'significant coronary disease'. And many patients have coronary artery bypass surgery without learning how to make a success of it. Returning autonomy to the patient is an essential part of rehabilitation, and can be very difficult when the patient expects a cure for the 'disease' or magic bullets for the symptoms of catabolic degradation.

Hyperventilation

The functions of the internal milieu and their orchestration are extremely sensitive to disturbances of the acid–base balance, and they cannot enjoy order and stability if the breathing is variable and excessive, blowing off too much carbon dioxide and causing alkalosis. The consequences can be slight if the person is in healthy function but devastating when he or she is robbed of homoeostatic, self-regulating power by extreme fatigue or exhaustion. The hyperventilation promotes arousal of the fight–flight (S-AM) mechanisms, and can put a powerful adrenergic jolt into the system. It causes anxiety, and urges the individual rightwards and downwards on the HFC, inhibiting anabolism and promoting catabolism. The effects, naturally enough, are widespread and every one of them is an obstacle to rehabilitation.

The skeletal muscles are subjected to cramp, pains and weakness (this is increased by the concomitant potassium loss); and the contraction of smooth muscle can cause such conditions as asthma, duodenal spasm and hiatus hernia, and spastic colon. The constriction of the muscular wall of blood vessels encourages hypertension, Raynaud's disease and allied peripheral disorders, and reduces the threshold for angina pectoris by congesting the heart and lungs as the great veins empty their reservoirs.

The heart is directly affected by hyperventilation, particularly through the increase of ionised calcium in its cells. Its wall may be stiffened and its chamber over-distended; its maintenance of orderly rhythm disturbed; and its blood flow reduced by spasm or constriction of the coronary arteries at a time when its demands are extravagantly increased by S-AM influences, and its ability to take up oxygen is reduced by the Bohr effect. The spasm and constriction can crack intimal plaques and damage the intimal lining of the coronary arteries, thereby creating great risk of thrombosis because the adrenergic drive and the changes of calcium metabolism increase the platelet-stickiness and the coagulability of the blood.

Even when the coronary arteries are normal these various results of hyperventilation can cause angina pectoris, myocardial infarction and sudden death; so crucial elements of cardiac rehabilitation are the management of the breathing and the elimination of the exhaustion that can enable hyperventilation to trigger disability and disaster.

For the purposes of rehabilitation, it should be assumed, until proved to the contrary, that cardiac neurosis and effort syndrome; unspecific conditions such as ME and post-viral syndrome; chest pain mimicking angina pectoris; and the illness behaviour found after open-heart surgery or admission into a coronary care unit are the products of exhaustion and hyperventilation.

Further accounts of the roles and relationships of hyperventilation can be found in the following references: Freeman and Nixon (1985a, b, 1987a); Nixon (1986b, c); Nixon and Freeman (1987a, b); Nixon, Freeman and King (1987); King (1988). Excellent general reviews are provided by Lum (1976) and Magarian (1982).

Destabilisation of the Cardiovascular System by Dynamic Factors

Atheroma is a middle-aged trait, and severe degrees of it may be found in active, healthy people: 'a man may get on very comfortably with practically a fourth of the whole system' (Osler, 1910). Bassler and Scaff (1976) have even trained a marathon runner who had 99, 95 and 80 per cent narrowings of his three major coronary arteries.

We tend to forget that the patterns of coronary atheroma found in angina pectoris are no different from those in people who seem to be healthy. The morbidity, and the mortality rates associated with angina pectoris are certainly not proportionate to the extent of the coronary atheroma (Sowton, 1979). Before the initial onset of symptoms there are long silent periods when the chronic arterial lesions do not interfere with daily life. Once symptoms have emerged they may disappear for several years, and the appearances and disappearances are not linked to detectable anatomical changes (Baroldi, Mariani and Falzi, 1978; Gorlin, 1976). It is common to find huge differences of effort tolerance, as much as 100-fold between 'good days' and 'bad days' in the earlier phases of angina pectoris, and these cannot be explained by any theory that postulates rigid, atheromatous stenosis as the sole cause of the pain and the disability (Maseri, 1980). Even in the case of sudden and unexpected death, pathologists are questioning whether the pathogenesis of the cardiac arrest has much to do with the chronic coronary artery lesions that are such a common finding in our culture (James, 1983). Except for the most extreme cases of coronary atheroma, in which rigid stenoses are unarguably and overwhelmingly dominant, it is clear that factors we call dynamic (Freeman and Nixon, 1985b) must play a leading part in the genesis of angina pectoris, myocardial infarction and sudden death, and be capable of producing these manifestations of internal disorder and destabilisation. The position is illustrated in Figure 4.

Medical science has not yet learned how to control the accumulation or regression of atheroma but surgical treatment and angioplasty are available as precise and logical responses to severe atherosclerotic narrowings. But they are costly, and reactive to the later stages of disease. What must be developed by cardiac rehabilitation are precise and logical responses to the dynamic factors (Nixon, 1986c; King and Nixon, 1988) that cause loss of order and stability in people who might be able to enjoy life and health without them.

I am convinced that the major dynamic factors are few in number, arousal-related, and generated by the behavioural and the neuroendocrine consequences of life on the down-slope of the HFC. They appear to be permutations and combinations of exhaustion and hyperventilation with heart injury produced by over-use and ischaemic battering. Contrary to popular medical opinion, the over-use and the battering with ischaemia are more often silent than painful (Freeman and Nixon, 1987a). Cardiac rehabilitation must accommodate this fact and teach it urgently, because most physicians acquiesce in harmful and self-defeating levels of activity if they are reported as painfree by patients, and many even encourage painful levels of activity without realising that the ischaemic damage is done before the pain is felt. The vasodilator prescribed might ease the pain but will not mend the damage already done, nor the accumulation of its effects.

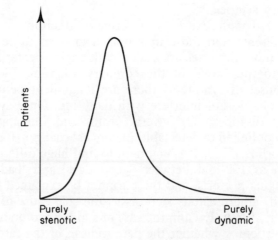

Figure 4   A model of a distribution curve for angina pectoris: it suggests that a few cases are caused by purely rigid atherosclerotic factors and a few by purely dynamic factors. The majority have both elements contributing to the symptoms.

The Scope, the Ethos and the Practice of Cardiac Rehabilitation

Cardiac rehabilitation is concerned with the people who are losers, for the moment, in the contest to maintain a stable and orderly internal milieu in an environment that is turbulent and uncertain, and generating arousal at an unprecedented rate (Figure 5). They are exhausted and wounded by the products of catabolism and hyperventilation, and suffering from the effects of a heart injured by over-use and ischaemic battering. The extent of coronary atheromatous handicap may be anything from trivial to an overwhelming severity that calls for urgent surgical treatment.

Reductionist treatment by risk factor modification and exercise prescription (Nixon, Al-Abbasi, King and Freeman, 1986) has not achieved very much so this chapter describes the problems in full, and in such a way as to invite other approaches. The field is open.

The heart is clearly subordinate to the brain and sensitive to the processes of the mind. At the same time, the processes of the mind and the coping ability are influenced by the individual's perception of his or her heart's condition. Thus it is logical to postulate that rehabilitation must accommodate both the problems of the mind and the heart and adopt a biopsychosocial model—competent clinical craftsmanship and an efficient technical service integrated with humane and compassionate relationships that respect the patient's dignity, sense of values and cultural canons. The cardiologist must work with the patient in a co-operative way, as a trainer; they must agree upon the objectives of therapy together, and make a joint effort to achieve them. The cardiologist must be sensitive to suffering and distress, and minimise the interventions that threaten the intactness of the individual and his or her relationships with other people. The cardiologist should be aware that the recovery of healthy function or adaptation to handicap may be impossible if medical interventions and the perception of illness make the patient incapable of occupying a satisfactory position in society. The care the cardiologist provides reduces the patient's need for vigilance that, like suffering and depersonalisation, can cause exhaustion and loss of resistance to disease. The cardiologist must pay close attention to the family, dealing as carefully as possible with their feelings of fear, anger and guilt. He or she must be aware of their hopes and anxieties, and reinforce their ability to deal with the heart-attacks in their midst. The biopsychosocial approach can accommodate the idea of angina pectoris and myocardial infarction as expressions of breakdown of the internal systems, and respond by integrating the best of contemporary technology with the best possible training for health, adaptation and coping (Cousins, 1983).

The processes of rehabilitation fall into three phases: stopping, resting and sleeping, and going back (Nixon, 1987).

Stopping

This is the difficult part. Exhausted patients driving themselves towards functional or organic failure of the heart do not want to give up the struggle

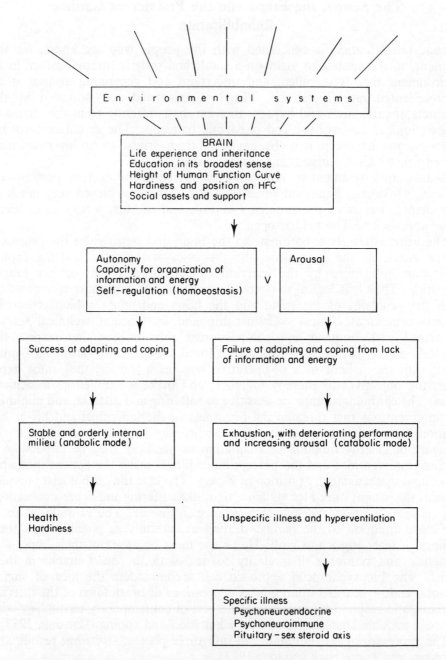

Figure 5   The contest for health and survival: individuals use their assets and pit their wills and skills against the potentially overwhelming influences of arousal. The outcome of failure or success is indicated.

to close the gap between their actual ability and their intentions. Denial and alexithymia make them oblivious of their position. Left cerebral hemispheric dominance (Henry, 1986) removes perspective and deafens them to the advice of the well-meaning. They can see no intermediate state between carrying on and 'becoming a cabbage'. Medical threats usually aggravate the intensity of the arousal and increase the risk. Palliative drugs are commonly sought and popularly prescribed for reducing symptoms without much attention being paid to the course of the contest with the environment.

Once the cardiologist has decided to confront the patient with the need to stop, the task of persuasion is probably best left to someone trained for this sort of crisis intervention. The purpose of stopping is to limit damage and provide the opportunity for recovery from exhaustion and homoeostatic disarray.

Resting and sleeping

The patient's role is passive here: accepting a rite of passage, a licence to withdraw from effort and vigilance in order to enjoy the rest and sleep that is required for the reduction of arousal and recovery of position on the up-slope of the HFC. The demands upon the heart and coronary circulation, and the catabolic disorders are reduced, and the anabolic opportunities expanded. The dynamic factors subside, autonomic stability is recovered, and the impact of hyperventilation is damped down. Homoeostasis can redevelop power.

The nurse is the person responsible for organising the therapeutic atmosphere in hospital or at home, for establishing a supportive relationship and using gifts of voice and touch to speed the recovery of order and stability. The nurse must be able to recognise and deal with hyperventilation and use sedation as required. The patient who accepts the need for sleep can achieve it, say, before and after lunch and at night by using small doses of promethazine hydrochloride and/or diazepam 5 mg under supervision. A salutary result can be hard to achieve if the patient is unwilling or the atmosphere disturbing, and so the personal influence of the nurse is a crucial matter. He or she must be able to deal with the presence of enormous levels of anger, and of fear masquerading as aggression without losing compassion and alienating the patient as a 'difficult' case. The patient must be conducted as quickly as possible through the phases of denial, rage and bargaining into the acceptance and awareness required for effective rehabilitation.

The resting-sleeping regimen (Nixon, 1973) is a practical, modern way of providing for our biological 'conservation-withdrawal' needs (Engel and Schmale, 1972). The recovery of a normal sleeping pattern and of the ability to adapt and habituate are essential ingredients.

The duration and intensity of the regimen varies, according to need, from a day in bed at home to a few days in hospital. It is commonly used prophylactically for the prevention of relapse into illness if exhaustion reappears in the later stages of rehabilitation. When patients begin to get up and about after myocardial infarction, the nurse teaches them to take their own pulse rate in order that they may use it to judge their own fitness for activity and recognise the limits of acceptable exertion.

Evans (1983) has studied the problems of early ambulation and premature discharge from hospital and written 'in complicated cases a walk around the ward on the twelfth day appears to do no harm, the patient having rested for a full nine days and remaining in care in hospital for 21 days, but THERE IS NO SOUND BASIS FOR EARLIER AMBULATION'. It is hard to achieve these standards in the NHS today.

Going back

In my department the occupational therapist (OT) meets patients during the passive phase. She can act as their advocate if they feel lost in the hospital system and assist them to settle down comfortably. It is her responsibility to assess what they require for going back to the activities of daily life in the best possible fashion.

The assessment takes account of the patients' assets and handicaps (high or low HFC) and of their intended levels of activity. Motivation and readiness for effort are weighed up in the knowledge that most urban families no longer know how to conduct illness. Domestic tension may be too high for convalescence or recovery to be feasible, and the spouse may need to be rested or eased into a more comfortable position for providing support. Hitherto rebellious children can turn out to be remarkably supportive if the crisis of the illness is well-used.

The assessment also takes account of the nursing process and the cardiological findings, and this calls for a close integration of effort with the medical team. The OT must also explore the patients' way of looking at the illness: a patient may have been so weary in the year before myocardial infarction that he or she has lost all hope of recovering healthy function. Jettisoning one activity after another (Nixon and Bethell, 1974) or wasting opportunities for recovery in fruitless attempts to do too much (Freeman and Nixon, 1987a; Nixon and Freeman, 1987b), patients usually rationalise their position as one of senility or incurable disease. It is the OT's job to act as a guide and trainer as each patient, weakened by pre-infarction ill-health and the impact of the illness, makes his or her way back into the contest with the environment. It is not intended that patients should simply return with attitudes unchanged to the same environmental influences that caused their breakdowns. It is assumed that they will want to learn how to go back to optimal activity at the best possible rate. There is much to be done. They must leave behind their patient status, recover autonomy and become highly informed people. They need to learn to use their self-organising abilities for defence and, if possible for the achievement of hardiness. They need to understand the strengths and weaknesses of their own homoeostatic system and provide what it requires for withstanding periods of high and prolonged arousal. If required, they must learn to adapt to handicap and make the best of it.

The essence of these needs is summarised by the acronym SABRES:

S = *Sleep*: awareness of the quantity and quality required, and how to get it.
A = *Arousal*: awareness. Learning to relax and modulate the effects of rage and struggle, despair and defeat well enough to keep out of catabolic disarray.
B = *Breathing*: awareness and control in place of hyperventilaton's upper-chest irregularities of rate and depth and sighing.
R = *Rest*: achieving the ability to be still and calm when the heart needs to be rested.
E = *Effort*: recognising and respecting the limits of beneficial physical and mental effort, and the onset of healthy tiredness.
S = *Self-esteem* and confidence: restored by the close support of the trainer and the successful employment of SABRE.

Descriptions of methods have been published elsewhere. I recommend Oswald and Adam (1983) for sleep, and Madders for techniques of relaxation in adults (1981), and children (1987). Lum (1976) on hyperventilation is unparalleled. The application of physical exercise may be found in Murray (1986) and Patel (1987). An account of occupational therapy in cardiac rehabilitation can be found in King (1987), King and Nixon (1988), and in hyperventilation in King (1988).

Cardiac rehabilitation requires a wide variety of skills and I have been fortunate enough to be able to call upon counsellors for crisis-intervention and family work, hypnotherapists, religious teachers, instructors in relaxation, masseuses, physiotherapists who practice massage, osteopaths, remedial gymnasts and dance therapists. Within the NHS most of them have given their services voluntarily, and so matters of agreement about standards and methods, supervision, the integration of activities and the exchanges of information at different levels might have created serious problems without the enterprise and co-ordinating ability of my colleague in OT, Jenny King. This work has provided an opportunity for practitioners in both complementary and conventional medicine to meet and learn about each other's language and attitudes.

Problems

The obstacles to the adoption of a systems or biopsychosocial approach to medicine and rehabilitation are legion. Our culture is oblivious of the fact that rest, sleep and withdrawal are biological imperatives. The rejection of paternalistic 'man-management' allows employees to be burned out and discarded. We have forgotten how to use our natural talents for healing and, once exhausted, we force ourselves downwards into illness and breakdown under ill-timed exhortations to change long-established diets, activities and habits when we have neither the mind for these tasks nor the will to succeed.

Even on the brink of a coronary breakdown, or when severely hypertensive from excessive and prolonged effort, we are incapable of going off-duty for recovery if the withdrawal lets others down—and it almost always does! We are not taught that both health and destiny can be influenced by the exercise of will, skilful self-organisation and the maintenance of a stable and orderly internal milieu.

Doctors are the product of the same culture, and they are no longer trained to deal with states of fatigue, exhaustion and unspecific illness induced by excessive and over-prolonged effort. They do not prescribe a period of withdrawal for sleeping and resting as a therapeutic test of the patient's ability to recover spontaneously, and they tend to be helpless—except for the prescription of drugs—and embarrassed when faced with patients in states of extremely high emotional arousal.

Many doctors are unable to distinguish between 'diseases' and stress-induced disturbances of the internal milieu, and are therefore inclined to treat them in the same way. The pharmaceutical industry makes a great profit from this reductionist approach to hypertension.

Medical education does not teach doctors ways of containing uncertainty. And so fruitless hunting for specific diagnosis and treatment can spoil the quality of a patient's life when that patient is exhausted, and remove the opportunity for rest and recovery by natural means.

The hyperventilation-related disorders do not appear in undergraduate textbooks today, and so severely handicapped patients can be given a dubious diagnosis such as 'post viral fatigue syndrome' or assured that there is 'nothing physically wrong'.

The patients themselves produce many problems. Some lack the information and do not get the leadership they require for harnessing the processes of recovery. Others move into denial of illness and responsibility for recovery. There are many reasons for denial. They include fear of the unknown and inability to grapple with the consequences of acceptance. Some put themselves 'above it all' because they do not want to entertain thoughts of weakness or imperfections: they may not wish to associate as fellow patients with damaged people. Others fight to the death to support a range of activities that has long since outstripped their resources.

Some patients fail because they want to keep up self-defeating levels of anger or indignation, and others because they cannot do without exhausting levels of displacement activity. Rehabilitation is probably wasted upon those whose deepest urge is to drop out of the rat-race and use a heart-attack or heart operation as a rite of passage into protected status: they are not likely to leave it just to please the doctor. It is equally wasted upon those who enjoy conflict and strive to neutralise their therapist's clinical skills with intellectual arguments.

Some failures of rehabilitation are due to helplessness and hopelessness: success, role-satisfaction and self-actualisation may be thought to be out of reach after the heart has been wounded. Others are due to an individual's inability to deal with a wound that cannot be seen, and to explain its implications to others. A great number fail because their households are too high in arousal to permit the natural processes of recovery.

It seems to me that the media are responsible for a great deal of failure because they parade the doctrines of the risk factor zealots without providing education for survival in a turbulent and uncertain social environment.

Successes

One Canadian study has reported a 47 per cent reduction of mortality in coronary patients through the provision of a nurse-counselling service (Frasure-Smith and Prince, 1985).

Our own 'randomised controlled trial to assess the effect of cardiac rehabilitation (using the Charing Cross model) in patients following myocardial infarction' enables the observers to compare biopsychosocial rehabilitation by occupational therapists with conventional medical treatment. The trial is half-way to completion and certain trends are emerging: it seems that the rehabilitation patients have less angina and a greater capacity for effort at three months; their illness behaviour appears to be less, and re-admissions to hospital fewer. Hyperventilation-related problems are reduced. The consumer reactions have not yet been measured, but most of the patients seem to be extremely pleased to have an OT as a guide and trainer, providing a personal service and access by telephone as compared with those treated conventionally through attendance at out-patient clinics (King and Nixon, 1988).

Ways Forward

There is so much to be done! Health education resources might be used to teach the systems approach and to make the public aware of the factors that are important for success and failure in the individual's never-ending contest with the turbulent and uncertain environment. Many people look upon an anabolic operating mode as a matter of common sense, and we need to be able to give them a licence to enjoy it instead of insisting that they move over the top of the HFC into illness and breakdown before management and medicine give attention to their needs. Too much attention is paid to medicine's responses to breakdown, and too little to the processes of anticipation and prevention, and the cultivation of hardiness. We should be aware of the importance of social assets, and think of more acceptable and helpful forms of social support for the vulnerable. The needs of the carers are neglected when provision is made for the sick.

Schoolchildren might be taught to relax and play as well as to compete in games, and they might also be taught something of what is learned in the martial arts, namely to be aware of the act of breathing in everyday life and to guard themselves against hyperventilation at times of exhaustion and distress.

Rehabilitation by occupational therapists is cheaper than the use of drugs to suppress the symptoms of the overloaded heart and the overtaxed mind, and I believe it reduces the need for coronary surgery. It enables us to integrate conventional, highly technological cardiology with the skills of complementary therapy. It seems to me that cost-effectiveness, skill-mix and quality of life considerations call for close co-operation between occupational therapists and heart specialists.

References

Adam, K., and Oswald, I. (1984) 'Sleep helps Healing'. *British Medical Journal*, **289**, 1400–1401.

Appels, A. (1983) 'The Year Before Myocardial Infarction', in Dembroski T.M., Schmidt, T.H. and Blümchen, G. (eds) *Biobehavioral bases of coronary heart disease*. Karger, Basel. p18–38.

Baroldi, G., Mariani, G., and Falzi, G. (1978) 'Degree of Coronary Obstruction at Autopsy in Patients with Coronary Heart Disease Compared with "Control Population"', In: Maseri, A., Klassen G.A., Lesch, M. (eds) Primary and Secondary Angina Pectoris. Grune & Stratton, New York.

Bassler, T., and Scaff, J. (1976) 'Marathon Runner'. *Lancet*, **2**, 544.

Beale, N., and Nethercott, S. (1986), 'Job Loss and Health—the Influence of Age and Previous Morbidity', *Journal of the Royal College of General Practitioners*, **36**, 261–264.

Berger, Y. (1987) 'Sea Pilots: the Problems of Extra Hours', *Seaways*, 7–10.

Bernard, C. (1867) In *Principles of General Physiology*. Longmans, London, (1960). p721–2.

British Medical Journal (1971) Editorial: 'The Murmuring Heart', **4**, 125–126.

British Medical Journal (1977) Editorial: 'Very Early Recognition of Coronary Heart Disease', **1**, 1302.

Buell, J. C., and Eliot, R. S. (1980) 'Psychosocial and Behavioral Influences in the Pathogenesis of Acquired Cardiovascular Disease', *American Heart Journal*, **100**, 723–740.

Cassell, J. (1976) 'The Contribution of the Social Environment to Host Resistance', *American Journal of Epidemiology*, **104**, 107–123.

Cousins, N. (1983), 'The Healing Heart'. *International Journal of Cardiology* **3** 57–65, 219–229.

Daily Telegraph (1983) 'Factory Workers at Greater Risk After Heart Advice', 14 May, p.15.

Dimsdale, J. E., and Herd, J. A. (1982) 'Variability of Plasma Lipids in Response to Emotional Arousal', *Psychosomatic Medicine*, **44**, 413–430.

Dubos, R. (1980) *Man Adapting*. Yale University Press.

Edwards, R. (1964) *Coronary Case*. Faber, London.

Engel, G. L., and Schmale, A. H.(1972) 'Physiology, Emotion and Psychosomatic Disease'. *Ciba Foundation, Symposium 8* (New series). Elsevier/ Excerpta Medica/ North-Holland, Amsterdam

Engel, G. L. (1974) Memorial Lecture: 'The Psychosomatic Approach to Individual Susceptibility to Disease', *Gastroenterology*, **67**, 1085–1093.

Engel, G. L. (1980) 'The Clinical Application of the Biopsychosocial Model' *American Journal of Psychiatry*, **137**, 535–544.

Engel, G. L. (1982). 'The Biopsychosocial Model and Medical Education', *New England Journal of Medicine*, **306**, 802–805.

Evans, D. W. (1983) 'Early Ambulation after Myocardial Infarction', *Journal of the Royal College of Physicians*, **17**, 217–219.

Eyer, J. (1980) 'Social Causes of Coronary Heart Disease', *Psychotherapy and Psychosomatics*, **34**, 75–87.

Farrant, W., and Russell, J. (1986) 'The Politics of Health Education', *Bedford Way Papers 28*. Institute of Education, University of London.

Frasure-Smith, N., and Prince, R. (1985) 'The Ischaemic Heart Disease Life Stress Monitoring Program: Impact on Mortality', *Psychosomatic Medicine* 47, 431–445.

Freeman, L. J., and Nixon, P. G. F. (1985a) 'Chest Pain and the Hyperventilation Syndrome—Some Aetiological Considerations', *Postgraduate Medical Journal* 61, 957–961.

Freeman, L. J. and Nixon, P. G. F. (1985b) 'Dynamic Causes of Angina Pectoris' *American Heart Journal* 110, 1087–1092.

Freeman, L. J., and Nixon, P. G. F. (1987a) 'Time to Rethink the Clinical Syndrome of Angina Pectoris?—Implications from Ambulatory ST Monitoring', *Quarterly Journal of Medicine*, 62 (237) 25–32.

Freeman, L. J., and Nixon, P. G. F. (1987b) 'Emotional State and Coronary Artery Disease: a Literature Review', *Holistic Medicine*, 2 145–154.

Friedman, M., and Rosenman, R. H. (1974) *Type A Behavior and Your Heart*. Wildwood House, London.

Gorlin, R., (1976). *Coronary Artery Disease*, p.179. W. B. Saunders, London.

Groen, J. J. (1976). 'Psychosomatic Aspects of Ischaemic (Coronary) Heart Disease', in Hill, O. (ed.) *Modern Trends in Psychosomatic Medicine* Vol. 3. Butterworth, London.

Gruzelier, J. H., Nixon, P. G. F., Liddiard, D., Pugh, S., and Baxter, R. (1986) 'Retarded Habituation and Lateral Asymmetries in Electrodermal Activity in Cardiovascular Disorders', *International Journal of Psychophysiology*, 3, 219–226.

Hebb, D. O. (1955) 'Drives and the C.N.S. (Conceptual Nervous System)', *Psychological Review*, 62, 243–254.

Henry, J. P. (1975). 'The Induction of Acute and Chronic Cardiovascular Disease in Animals by Psychosocial Stimulation', *International Journal of Psychiatric Medicine*, 6, 147–158.

Henry, J. P. (1982) 'The Relation of Social to Biological Processes in Disease', *Social Science and Medicine*, 16, 369–380.

Henry, J. P. (1986) 'Mechanisms by Which Stress Can Lead to Coronary Heart Disease', *Postgraduate Medical Journal*, 62, 687–693.

Henry, J. P. (1987) 'Psychological Factors and Coronary Heart Disease'. *Holistic Medicine*, 2, 119–132.

Henry, J. P., and Meehan, J. P. (1981) 'Psychosocial Stimuli, Physiological Specificity, and Cardiovascular Disease, in: Weiner, H., Hofer, M.A., and Stunkard, A.J. (eds). *Brain, Behavior and Bodily Disease*. Raven Press, New York.

Henry, J. P., and Stephens, P. M.(1977) '*Stress, Health, and the Social Environment*. Springer, New York.

Hilton, J. (1863) *On the Influence of Mechanical and Physiological Rest*. Bell & Daldy, London.

Journal of the American Medical Association (1982) 'Multiple Risk Factor Intervention Trial Research Group', 248, 1465–1477.

James, T. N. (1983) 'Chance and Sudden Death'. *Journal of the American College of Cardiologists*, 1, 164–183.

Jenkins, C. D. (1978) 'Low Education: a Risk Factor for Death', *New England Journal of Medicine*, 299, 95–97.

Jenkins, C. D., Stanton, B. E., Klein, M. D., Savageau, J. A., and Harken, D. E. (1983) 'Correlates of Angina Pectoris Among Men Awaiting Coronary Artery By-pass Surgery', *Psychosomatic Medicine*, 45, 141–153.

Johnson, A. (1977) 'Sex Differentials in Coronary Heart Disease: the Explanatory Role of Primary Risk Factors', *Journal of Health and Social Behavior*, **18**, 46–54.

Kagan, A. (1982) 'Introduction to the Role of Psychosocial Stressors in Ischaemic Heart Disease,' In Kellerman (ed).*Psychological Problems Before and After Myocardial Infarction*. Karger, Basel.

Kagan, A., and Levi, L. (1974) 'Health and Environment—Psychosocial Stimuli: a Review' *Social Science and Medicine* **8**, 225–241.

Kahnemann, D. (1973) *'Attention and Effort'*, Prentice-Hall, Englewood Cliffs, NJ.

Karasek, R. A., Russell, S. R., and Theorell, T. (1982) 'Physiology of Stress and Regeneration in Job Related Cardiovascular Illness', *Journal of Human Stress*, **8**, 29–42.

King, J. C. (1987) 'Coronary Care'. In: Turner, A. (ed.) *The Practice of Occupational Therapy*. Churchill-Livingstone, London.

King, J. C. (1988) 'Hyperventilation—A Therapist's Point of View', *Journal of the Royal Society of Medicine*, **81**, 532–536.

King, J. C., Nixon P. G. F. (1988) A system of Cardiac Rehabilitation: Psychophysiological Basis and Practice, Br. J. Occup. Ther. **51**, 378–384.

Knutsson, A., Akerstedt, T., Jonsson, B. G., and Örth-Gomer, K. (1986) 'Increased Risk of Ischaemic Heart Disease in Shift Workers', *Lancet*, **ii**, 89–92.

Kobasa, S. C., Maddi, S. R., and Kahn, S. (1982) 'Hardiness and Health: a Prospective Study', *Journal of Personality and Social Psychology*, **42**, 168–177.

Koestler, A. (1978) *Janus: A Summing Up*. Hutchinson, London.

Kringlen, E. (1986) 'Psychosocial Aspects of Coronary Heart Disease', *Acta Psychiatrica Scandinavica* **74**, 225–237.

Lader, M. (1975) In: Levi, L. (ed.) *Emotions, Their Parameters and Measurement*, p.361. Raven Press, New York.

Lane, R. D., and Schwartz, G. E. (1987) 'Induction of Lateralised Sympathetic Input to the Heart by the C.N.S. During Emotional Arousal: a Possible Neurophysiologic Trigger of Sudden Cardiac Death', *Psychomsomatic Medicine*, **49**, 274–284.

Levi, L. (1972) *'Stress and Distress in Response to Psychosocial Stimuli'*, Pergamon Press, Oxford.

Lipowski, Z. J. (1975) 'Sensory and Information Inputs Overload: Behavioural Effects', *Comprehensive Psychiatry*, **16**, 199–221.

Lorenz, K. (1970) *'On Aggression'* Methuen, University Paperback Edition, London.

Lown, B., DeSilva, R., Reich, P., and Murawski, B. J. (1980) 'Psychophysiologic Factors in Sudden Cardiac Death', *American Journal of Psychology* **137**, 1325–1335.

Lum, L. C. (1976) 'The Syndrome of Habitual Chronic Hyperventilation' In Hill, O. W. (ed.) *Modern Trends in Psychosomatic Medicine*, **Vol. 3**. Butterworths, London.

Lynch, J. J. (1977). *The Broken Heart: The Medical Consequences of Loneliness*. Basic Books, New York.

Madders, J. (1981) *Stress and Relaxation*, Hay, M. (ed.). Positive Health Guide, Martin Dunitz, London.

Madders, J. (1987). *Relax and be Happy*. Unwin, London.

Magarian, G. J. (1982) 'Hyperventilation Syndromes: Infrequently Recognised Common Expressions of Anxiety and Stress', *Medicine*, **61**, 219–236.

Malliani, A. (1982) 'Cardiovascular Sympathetic Afferent Fibers', *Reviews in Physiology, Biochemistry and Pharmacology*, **94**, 11–74.

Maseri, A. (1980) 'Pathogenetic Mechanisms of Angina Pectoris: Expanding Views', *British Heart Journal*, **43**, 648–660.

McKeigue, P. M., Marmot, M. G., Adelstein, A. M., Hunt, S. P., *et al.* (1985) 'Diet and Risk Factors for Coronary Heart Disease in Asians in Northwest London', *Lancet*, **ii**, 1086–1090.

Metcalfe, D. H. H. (1981) 'The Role of Patient Participation in the Development of Rational Health Services'. *Journal of the Royal College of General Practitioners*, Occasional paper 17, pp.1–2.

Miettinen, T. A., Huttunen, J. K., Naukkarinen, V., Strandberg, T. *et al.* (1985) 'Multifactorial Primary Prevention of Cardiovascular Diseases in Middle-aged Men', *Cardiovascular Diseases*, **254**, 2097.

Mitchell, J. R. A. (1984) 'What Constitutes Evidence on the Dietary Prevention of Coronary Heart Disease? Cosy Beliefs or Harsh Facts?', *International Journal of Cardiology*, **5**, 287–298.

Montagu, A. (1971) *Touching: The Human Significance of the Skin*. Columbia University Press, New York.

Montagu, A. (1976) *The Nature of Human Aggression*. Oxford University Press, London.

Murray, A. (1986). *Return to Fitness*. Batsford, London.

Myers, A., and Dewar, H. A. (1975) 'Circumstances Attending 100 Sudden Deaths from Coronary Artery Disease with Coroner's Necropsies', *British Heart Journal*, **37**, 1133–1143.

Nixon, P. G. F. (1973) 'Coronary Heart Disease and its Emergencies', *Practitioner*, **35**, 1–12.

Nixon, P. G. F. (1976) 'The Human Function Curve', *Practitioner*, **217**, 765–769, 935–944.

Nixon, P. G. F. (1980) 'The Responsibility of the Cardiological Mapmaker', *American Heart Journal*, **100**, 139–143.

Nixon, P. G. F. (1982a) 'Stress and the Cardiovascular System', *Practitioner*, **226**, 1589–1598.

Nixon, P. G. F. (1982b) 'Are there Clinically Significant Prodromal Signs and Symptoms of Impending Sudden Death', *Practical Cardiology*, **8**, 175–183.

Nixon, P. G. F. (1984) 'Stress, Life Style and Cardiovascular Disease. A Cardiological Odyssey', *British Journal of Holistic Medicine* **1**, 20–29.

Nixon, P. G. F. (1986a) 'Does Stress Cause Heart Attacks? Psychosocial Factors in C.H.D', *The Coronary Prevention Group. Proceedings of a Conference*, 18–19 November 1985, p. 45–55.

Nixon, P. G. F. (1986b) 'Exhaustion: Cardiac Rehabilitation's Starting Point', *Physiotherapy*, **72**, 224–228.

Nixon, P. G. F. (1986c) 'Consensus Meeting: Coronary Artery Bypass Surgery—Is It Enough?'. *Quality of Life and Cardiovascular Care*, **2**, 125–132.

Nixon, P. G. F. (1987). 'Behavioral Management and Rehabilitation after Acute Myocardial Infarction', in *International Perspectives in Behavioral Medicine* (in press).

Nixon, P. G. F., and Bethell, H. N. (1974). 'Pre-Infarction Ill-Health', *American Journal of Cardiology*, **33**, 446–449.

Nixon, P. G. F., and Freeman, L. J. (1987a) 'The "think test": a further technique to elicit hyperventilation'. *Journal of the Royal Society of Medicine*, **81**, 277–279.

Nixon, P. G. F., and Freeman, L. J. (1987b) 'What Is the Meaning of Angina Pectoris Today?' *American Heart Journal* **114**, 1542–1546.

Nixon, P. G. F., Freeman, L. J. and King, J. C. (1987) 'Breathing and Thinking: Unacknowledged Coronary Risk Factors'. *Holistic Medicine*, **2**, 133–136.

Nixon, P. G. F., Al-Abbasi, A. H., King, J. C., and Freeman, L. J. (1986) 'Hyperventilation in Cardiac Rehabilitation', *Holistic Medicine*, **1**, 5–13.

Osler, W. (1910) 'Angina Pectoris', *Lancet*, **i**, 839.

Oswald, I., and Adam, K. (1983). *Get a Better Night's Sleep*. Positive Health Guide, Martin Dunitz, London.

Patel, C. (1987) *Fighting Heart Disease*. Pietroni P. (ed.). Dorling Kindersley, London.

Raab, W. (1969) 'Myocardial electrolyte derangement: crucial feature of pluricausal, so-called coronary heart disease', *Annals of the New York Academy of Sciences*, **147**, 627–686.

Rahe R. H., and Ransom, J A. (1978) 'Life Change and Illness Studies: and Future Directions', *Journal of Human Stress*, **4**, 3–15.

Ruberman, W., Weinblatt, E., Goldberg, J.D., and Chaudhary, B. S. (1984) 'Psychosocial Influences on Mortality after Myocardial Infarction', *New England Journal of Medicine*, **311**, 552–559.

Salonen, J. T. (1987) 'Did the North Karelia Project Reduce Coronary Mortality?', *Lancet*, **ii**, 269.

Siegrist, J. (1980) 'Cardiovascular Disease and the Sympathetic Nervous System', *Lancet*, **ii**, 1196.

Siegrist, J., Dittman, K., Rittner, K., and Weber, I. (1982) 'The Social Context of Active Distress in Patients with Early Myocardial Infarction', *Social Science and Medicine*, **16**, 443–453.

Sowton, E. (1979) 'The Treatment of Angina Pectoris', *Practitioner*, **223**, 471–476.

Sterling, P., and Eyer, J. (1981) 'Biological Basis of Stress-Related Mortality', *Social Science and Medicine*, **15E**, 3–42.

Sutherland, J. D. (1971) 'Stress and Society', In Bouchier, I. D. A. (ed.). *Seventh Symposium on Advanced Medicine*, p.155. Pitman Medical, London.

Tuchman, B. (1980) *The Proud Tower*, Macmillan, London.

Verrier, R. L., Hagestad, E.L., and Lown, B. (1987) 'Delayed Myocardial Ischaemia Induced by Anger', *Circulation*, **75**, 249–254.

Weiss, J. M. (1972) 'Influence of Psychological Variables on Stress-Induced Pathology', In *Physiology, Emotions and Psychosomatic Illness*. Ciba Foundation, Symposium 8, Elsevier-Excertpa Medica, Amsterdam.

Zwingmann, C. (1977) *Uprooting and Related Phenomena*. World Health Organisation, Geneva.

Glossary

Tracheostomy   The surgical formation of an opening into the trachea or windpipe at the root of the neck, formerly carried out when artificial respiration by machine was required for more than a matter of hours.

Metabolic acidosis and alkalosis   Loss of the normal acid/alkali equilibrium of the body in a shift towards one extreme or the other.

Heart block   An abnormally low heart rate caused by interference with the heart's electrical system.

Arrhythmias   Disturbances of the heart's normal rhythm of beating.

Low cardiac output conditions   Inability of the heart, from any of a variety of causes, to pump enough blood for the needs of the body and for its own nourishment, as, for example, in the state of shock.

Heart catheterisation   The insertion of plastic tubes or catheters into the heart in order to make accurate diagnoses. The chambers of the right side of the heart can be entered by catheters introduced into a vein in one of the limbs, but the lungs prevent onward passage to the left atrium and left ventricle. The left atrium was reached in the early days by a needle passed upwards through the venous system from the groin.

The catheter and needles allowed blood samples to be taken, pressures to be recorded, and dyes to be injected. These were opaque to X-rays and allowed films to be taken (angiography). Alternatively, materials such as hydrogen, ascorbic acid or blue dye could be introduced into the blood stream and their passage recorded by strategically placed sensors (indicator–dilution curves).

These techniques made it possible to assess the size and position of openings and conduits that shunted blood to abnormal destinations and interfered with the proper pressure relationships between different chambers of the heart. They also made it possible to distinguish abnormal narrowing of heart valves (stenosis) from states of abnormal widening with leakage (incompetence). Many fruitless operations for mitral stenosis were carried out before we learned that a noise called an opening snap, made by the diseased mitral valve, was not diagnostic of narrowing but could also occur in incompetence whose treatment involved the use of a heart–lung machine, a much more complicated operation. In incompetence, it indicated a form of incompetence that might be repaired without recourse to an artificial heart valve in the days before these prostheses were satisfactorily developed.

Homoeostasis   The body's capacity for maintaining a stable and orderly internal milieu in the face of varying external conditions.

Myocardial infarction, cardiac infarction   A portion of the heart muscle dying because its blood supply is cut off. In some cases a form of shock ensues that can be treated by the infusion of fluids because the blood volume becomes too low for the needs of the damaged heart (hypovolaemic cardiogenic shock).

Coronary insufficiency   Inadequacy of the coronary blood flow carrying ·the threat of infarction, and caused usually by constriction, spasm, or thrombosis of the artery at the site of disease (atheroma).

Angina pectoris   Pain caused by transient inadequacy of coronary blood flow from constriction or spasm and/or disease (atheroma).

Changing Ideas in Health Care
Edited by D. Seedhouse and A. Cribb
© 1989 John Wiley & Sons Ltd

Chapter Three
Changing the Agenda: The Role of the Cancer Self-Help Group

ANNE EARDLEY
Department of Epidemiology and Social Oncology
University of Manchester
UK

Introduction

Until recently, the suggestion that there was any scope for self-help among cancer patients would have seemed bizarre in the extreme. The enduring image of cancer is of a deadly, powerful disease, all too often impervious to medical intervention. However, in the last decade there has been such a dramatic growth in the number of self-help organisations for sufferers of a variety of conditions, including cancer, that the editor of the *British Medical Journal* has asserted that self-help groups should be recognised as the 'fourth estate' in medicine (Lock, 1986). The aim of this chapter is to assess the role of self-help organisations in cancer. To this end, it is necessary to describe the needs of people coping with cancer and the extent to which those needs are currently addressed by conventional health services. The chapter ends with a description of the activities of cancer self-help groups in general, and a detailed account of how one such group operates.

What Are the Needs of Those with Cancer?

An enormous volume of research into the psychosocial impact of cancer has been built up over the last three decades. The amount of research interest is itself an indicator that cancer is regarded as different from other diseases. At one level this can be understood with reference to Sontag's (1979) analysis: in Western societies, cancer is a metaphor for death and destruction, mysterious and uncontrollable; cancer fills the role once occupied by tuberculosis. Empirical support for this view of cancer comes from surveys of knowledge and opinions of cancer among the general public (Davidson, 1984; Knopf, 1976). There is a consistent tendency for people to overestimate the importance of cancer as a cause of death, and underestimate the extent to which it can be cured. Although there has been a steady increase in openness about cancer, both in terms of doctors' willingness to disclose the diagnosis to patients and in terms of public discussion about the disease, it is still common to see the words 'died after a long illness' in newspaper notices of death.

So the newly diagnosed person with cancer may have a frightening image of his or her disease. To this fear may be added uncertainty: uncertainty about the treatment that may be received [for example, misconceptions about radiotherapy are common (Eardley, 1986)] and about how effective it will be. As Peters-Golden (1982) pointed out in her study of breast cancer patients' perceptions of social support, 'cancer is different, not only because it fails to conform to the Western model of (known) cause and (predictable) effect, but also because even if the patient co-operates fully with the physician and follows the treatment regimen faithfully, there can be no guarantee that therapy will succeed'. Cancer treatments may in themselves cause additional stress, both in the short term and the long term: surgery, radiotherapy and chemotherapy all carry significant morbidity in terms of unpleasant physical side-effects and in some cases, for example, after radical surgery, permanent dysfunction or disfigurement. Emotional distress such as depression and anxiety may also be experienced and may persist for long periods. Maguire et al., (1978) found that no fewer than one in four women had moderate or severe depression, or anxiety, or both, one year after mastectomy.

In terms of life changes, there is a plethora of evidence suggesting that the experience of having cancer and undergoing treatment for cancer can have a marked impact on various important areas of life: work, social life, marital and family life (Feldman, 1978; Eardley et al., 1976; Follick, Smith and Turk, 1984; Rieker, Edbril and Garnick, 1985; Fobair et al., 1986). In part this may be a consequence of physical problems and limitations but these may be compounded by the psychological impact of a life-threatening disease with uncertain prognosis, and by the reactions of others: it is not uncommon for people with cancer to experience awkwardness, if not outright rejection, in dealings with relatives, friends and acquaintances. Peters-Golden (1982) found that 72 per cent of the women with breast cancer in her study reported that they were treated differently after people discovered that they had cancer. Often, the responses of others were unhelpful: 72 per cent of patients felt that they were misunderstood, and 52 per cent that they were avoided or feared: 60 per cent were made to feel separated and alone by unrelenting optimism, such as exhortations to 'cheer up'. The veracity of these accounts was confirmed in another part of the same survey, in which members of the public were asked about their attitudes towards people with cancer: 56 per cent said that they would avoid contact with someone they knew had cancer, and only 28 per cent said that they made no special effort to 'cheer up' a cancer patient or exhibit optimism in their presence. Evidence of this type throws some light on the reasons why people with cancer may feel that they are left to bear the 'burden of cancer' alone (Hinton, 1973).

To summarise: people with cancer have the task of coping with a stigmatised illness with uncertain prognosis; they must also cope with therapy that they do not fully understand, and which may have unpleasant after-effects. As with other serious illnesses, physical limitations imposed by the treatment or by the disease itself can lead to dependence upon others. In addition, the person's concept of the wholeness and health of their own body can be altered in the face of what is seen as an all-powerful and possibly fatal disease. Finally, the reactions of others may further undermine the cancer patient's feelings of self-worth.

How Are the Needs of Those with Cancer Met by Conventional Health Services?

In coping with the stresses of cancer, the patient may well be handicapped by feelings of powerlessness. In part these derive from the pervasive image of cancer as a disease over which one has little control, as well as from the physical assault of the disease and its therapies. But it is possible to argue that aspects of the organisation of conventional health care services do little to combat such feelings, and may indeed exacerbate them.

The situation of most people with cancer approximates closely to the traditional patient role: patients diagnosed with a potentially life-threatening disease are unlikely to do other than defer to the doctor's superior knowledge, and 'compliance' in the form of accepting or continuing what may be excessively toxic treatments is surprisingly high. Where the handling of cancer patients may differ from that of other patients is, if anything, in the direction of decreasing personal autonomy. Perhaps because health professionals are aware of the general public's image of cancer as a uniquely frightening disease, there may be a conspiracy of silence to protect patients from knowing their diagnosis and prognosis; certainly the volume of discussion in medical and research journals about communicating with the cancer patient is not replicated with other patient groupings. Although care in the choice of the amount of information a health professional imparts may be commended in principle, in practice it can reflect a stereotyping of the cancer patient as peculiarly fragile—someone who might 'go to pieces' in the face of bad news.

There is little in the organisation of any of the cancer therapies which either requires or promotes patient autonomy. Unlike patients with certain medical conditions (such as diabetes), cancer patients are not actively involved in their treatment, but are passive acceptors of it. Perhaps because active participation in treatment is not a prerequisite of effectiveness (all the patient has to do is to attend for treatment) professional attempts to increase patients' knowledge and understanding of their treatment and their disease are rare. Some hospitals have booklets available about particular types of treatment, but responsibility for their distribution is often inadequate, with the result that many patients receive nothing about their illness or their treatment in writing. Some specialist nurses have beeen appointed who can advise particular groups of patients, but the majority of patients are not covered by such a service.

Obtaining information is one way of establishing some measure of control over potentially frightening events. Ironically, it was a doctor with cancer who set up the first national cancer information service in Britain. In her account of how this service was established, Vicky Clement-Jones describes how she was struck by the great need for information among patients and their families.

At the same time, her own privileged position as a doctor gave her access to medical information which she felt 'contributed significantly to my quality of life' (Clement-Jones, 1985). She also recognised that practical information, such as how to cope with unpleasant side-effects of cancer treatment was not always forthcoming from professionals, but that patients themselves had a 'vast wealth of experience I felt was not being tapped effectively'.

The experience of this cancer patient illustrates a fundamental problem in the organisation of cancer services. As Houlton (1987) has pointed out, cancer is often regarded as an acute illness, and services are centred primarily around hospitals. Yet for the majority of cancer patients, cancer is 'a chronic disease with perhaps many periods of acute exacerbation'. As a percentage of the patient's total 'career', time spent at hospitals represents a tiny fraction, and much of the distress occasioned by treatment reactions, for example, will be endured at home. Contact between patient and professional is often brief and confined to an assessment of the patient's physical state. It is not usual for patients to be asked by health professionals to describe how they coped with the range of problems that they have had to face since their cancer was diagnosed. Such a fund of knowledge is an untapped resource, of particular relevance in the case of a chronic illness like cancer which brings with it many 'adaptive tasks' to be faced over a considerable period of time. Recognition within the health service that the cancer patient is a sentient being whose experiences could provide insight into the stresses occasioned by cancer would help to create a service more in tune with patients' needs and could also enhance patients' own feelings of self-worth.

The Role of the Cancer Self-Help Group

In a thoughtful analysis of the effect of cancer on the patient's interpersonal relationships, Wortman and Dunkel-Schetter (1979) maintain that 'because of the uncertainties they face and because their sense of self is threatened, many cancer patients experience intense needs, both to clarify what is happening to them and to be supported and reassured by others'. They describe various ways in which such needs can be met—by meeting others in a similar situation, by discussing one's feelings with a sympathetic listener, and by obtaining feedback about the meaning and appropriateness about such feelings. As already indicated, the likelihood of such needs being met within conventional health services is slight, but all of these functions may be fulfilled by lay people with personal experience of cancer. In an 'inside view' of cancer self-help groups, Tom Brown and Petra Griffiths, both cancer sufferers, describe the range of activities that might be undertaken: group meetings, telephone help lines, home and hospital visiting, practical help, and (rarely) residential care (Brown and Griffiths, 1986). Groups can vary in other ways: some have strong links with health professionals, and indeed some have been established by professionals. Others have been set up expressly to promote complementary therapies, and may have little if any contact with orthodox health practitioners.

The Example of CALL

Cancer Aid and Listening Line (CALL) was started in 1982 by a former cancer sufferer who had been diagnosed several years previously with Hodgkin's disease—a cancer affecting the lymph glands. He had made an excellent recovery, but at considerable personal cost—the illness and treatment having resulted in major changes in his life. It was this contrast between the effectiveness of the physical treatment of the disease and the seemingly complete absence of support for him as an individual coping with a life-threatening illness and its gruelling therapy that led him to believe that there was some deficiency in the service then offered to people with cancer.

The main impetus in setting up CALL was to offer emotional support to those affected by cancer. Given the limited resources of CALL in its initial stages, both in terms of money and in terms of the amount of personal time and energy that the small group of founder members of CALL could offer, it was felt that the most that could be managed at the outset was a meeting once a month, open to anyone affected by or interested in the problems caused by cancer. A room was offered, free of charge, by the local Health Education Officer, and meetings have continued to be held monthly ever since.

A format for meetings was established that has changed little in subsequent years. As people arrive they are offered tea and, in fact, it is deliberate policy to allow an informal period for chatting before the formal part of the meeting begins. It is standard for the meeting to be opened by the chairperson or a long-standing member of CALL. Seating is informal, but tends to be in a circle rather than in rows: the chairperson introduces him or herself, usually adding a few words about his or her own connection with cancer and about what CALL can offer. This is directed primarily at people attending a meeting for the first time, with the aim of putting them at their ease and recognising that their first attendance may not be easy. Those attending are then invited to introduce themselves; as they go round the circle, most people give only their name, but more established members may add a little about their connections with CALL; for example, that they are on the committee or that they have been coming since the group started. After any announcements, a speaker is introduced. Originally, every meeting had a speaker, but it was felt by committee members that people's need to talk was the main impetus to their attending, so in the last year or so, some meetings have been purely social, with no speaker. Speakers may be health professionals, for example, a doctor, radiographer or medical social worker talking about their work. Or they may be people with personal experience of cancer, telling their 'story'. More recently, the range of speakers has been extended to include people with an interest in complementary therapies for cancer, such as meditation.

The talk is followed by questions, and the final part of the evening is again informal. During this period, established members of CALL try to ensure that people attending for the first time and those with particular needs for either support or information are put in touch with someone who can help. This process is facilitated by the fact that CALL meetings are usually attended by a sprinkling of 'resource' people: some are professionals, such as nurses or social workers, others are CALL telephone volunteers who have not only been trained in listening skills, but also have information about the range of services available to people with cancer.

It had been envisaged at an early stage of CALL's existence that its service could be effectively extended if a telephone help-line were offered. Soon after the monthly meetings had been established, plans were made to set this up: volunteers were recruited with the help of a local newspaper article, and a training course was set up, run by a consultant psychiatrist who gave his time voluntarily. The aim of the course was not to produce trained counsellors: it was generally felt by the original CALL committee that the principle of self-help could be compromised if there were too big a difference between volunteers and those approaching CALL for help. On the other hand, they recognised the need to avoid the pitfalls that await the completely untrained volunteer: over-identification, and the failure to pick up pressing concerns. So the training set out to provide volunteers with some insight into the range of reactions to cancer, and to equip them with basic listening skills. The course had a practical component too: information about statutory and voluntary services for people with cancer was given, as was the opportunity to meet a selection of professionals involved in the care of cancer patients.

Since the first course, four more courses have been run for new telephone volunteers: the format of the course has not changed substantially, but the practical component was enlarged after the first course by adding a session giving basic information about cancer and its treatment. Initially there was some debate about the need for this, as there had always been a strong resistance among committee members to the idea of giving medical advice— in part because it was not seen as part of CALL's brief, but also because of the fear of antagonising health professionals and running the risk of compromising the good name of the group. However, it was finally agreed that it would be useful to provide background information to would-be volunteers, so that they would not be in a position whereby they did not understand terms used by callers.

From the beginning, the telephone line has operated in the following way: the line is open every evening, including weekends and public holidays, for a three-hour period. CALL publicity material provides a telephone number that gives a recorded message, providing the home telephone number of the volunteer for that evening. The decision to organise the service in this way was in part determined by circumstances: until recently, CALL had no premises of its own where volunteers could come to take calls. In addition, due to the geographical spread of volunteers, travelling regularly to a central venue would be an extra burden. In the event, initial fears that callers might abuse the service by repeatedly calling the same volunteer have not materialised, and out-of-hours calls are relatively uncommon.

The type of call made to the help-line covers a wide range of problems: an analysis of the first 100 calls received when the service began (Eardley and Brown, 1985) showed that relatives or friends of people with cancer were more likely to use the service than were people with cancer themselves; and that one of the most common topics that people wanted to discuss was the care of a person who was terminally ill. Problems described by callers facing this situation included lack of awareness of available services, exhaustion brought on by caring for the dying person unaided, concern over lack of symptom control and dilemmas over whether to tell the person 'the truth' about their situation. It is not uncommon for people making the calls to be deeply distressed: they may cry, or be so depressed as to find speaking difficult. Only very occasionally are they aggressive or abusive to the CALL volunteer.

To help volunteers cope with difficult or distressing calls, various support systems have been established. The main method of giving support is the monthly support meeting for telephone volunteers. At these meetings, calls are discussed by the volunteers as a group; individuals describing difficult calls are encouraged to report how they felt about the way they handled the call, and other members of the group give their opinions of how they felt the volunteer responded. Occasionally, a professional counsellor is invited to these meetings, to comment on particular calls and suggest ways of handling particularly difficult callers or problems.

It is also necessary to make provision for immediate support for volunteers between meetings; for example, when a call has been taken about which the volunteer feels disturbed. When this happens, volunteers are encouraged to telephone an experienced telephone volunteer straight away, so that some of the burden can be shared. Sometimes volunteers find a call difficult because it strikes a painful chord in their memory of their own experience; more commonly it is because the volunteer herself (a majority of volunteers are women, as are callers) feels inadequate in what she can offer. This may be because the caller is in such extreme distress that it is difficult for the volunteer to establish helpful contact. Or the caller may be in what seems an impossible position, for example, coping unaided with a dying relative, and on bad terms with the GP (usually the gatekeeper to other services). Alternatively, the caller may ask for something the volunteer cannot give; for example a home visit.*

CALL was able to expand its activities as a result of a grant obtained from the county council in 1985 that enabled the organisation to acquire premises and employ a part-time co-ordinator. One immediate expansion was in the phone-line service, which could now be offered during the daytime. A further development in the service offered was a drop-in facility: callers could now visit the centre to talk to the co-ordinator or one of the other trained volunteers if they preferred face-to-face contact to the anonymity of the phone line. Finally, there has been an increase in the number of activities or events in which members can participate; for example, a variety of people offering complementary methods of coping with cancer visit the centre to teach techniques of meditation and yoga.

An Assessment of the Role of Cancer Self-Help Groups

CALL has many features in common with other cancer self-help groups. Perhaps its main distinguishing features are the well-established telephone

---

*CALL has established a home visiting service in one of the health districts of Greater Manchester, using trained volunteers to support those caring for someone with cancer.

help-line and its neutral stance with regard to conventional medicine and complementary therapies alike, endorsing neither uncritically, but prepared to draw on the resources of both. Although it is not possible to assess with any degree of certainty how effectively cancer self-help groups such as CALL meet needs that are currently unmet, or inadequately met, by conventional health services, it is possible to describe the ways in which such groups might be well placed to meet those needs—the re-establishment of personal autonomy, the coming to terms with uncertainty, the coping with the physical consequences of cancer therapies and the disease itself.

The fact that it is composed of people with personal experience of cancer, either in themselves or in those close to them, *and* that those directly involved in giving a service such as the telephone line are trained to do so means that several unique opportunities present themselves. First, as with all self-help groups, CALL utilises the unique contribution of fellow-patients: those who have undergone similar experiences and who can, as a result, offer a type of reassurance and encouragement that is denied to those without that personal experience. (This is not to discount the reassurance that health professionals can offer, which comes from a different perspective and derives from experience of treating a large number of patients). Meeting a variety of people with experience of cancer provides examples of a range of 'coping styles', and helps to combat feelings of isolation: in talking to other cancer sufferers, it soon becomes apparent that one is not alone in one's experience of cancer-related problems. Furthermore, many of those utilising the services provided by CALL have spoken of their relief in being able to discuss their concerns openly without fear of upsetting relatives and friends. Conversely, for relatives and friends themselves an anonymous and neutral telephone service can provide a 'safety-valve' for those under stress from someone else's cancer that is not readily available elsewhere.

In addition, for groups with good, informal links with professionals, practical 'inside information' as to how to get the best from cancer services is available. Soon after the telephone link was established, it became apparent to telephone volunteers that knowledge of the services that existed for cancer patients was not enough; it was also necessary to know how to obtain them and how to get the most out of them. For example, it is one thing to know that hospices have expert knowledge on the control of pain: it is quite another to know how to 'tap in' to that expertise in the face of resistance from the patient's GP. Because of CALL's 'moderate' stance it has easy access to a range of health professionals as well as to 'experienced' members who can advise on problems such as these.

Informal contact with health professionals brings other benefits too; monthly meetings give those attending a unique opportunity to cross-question health professionals (attending either as speakers or informally) in what is hoped is a non-threatening environment—away from health services premises, and in the company of other lay people. In this atmosphere, patients and relatives may build up confidence in asking questions, and may also gain insight into some of the constraints operating on health professionals.

This leads on to a final consideration. CALL and other similarly constituted groups offer those health professionals interested enough to establish contact with the group, insights into the experience of coping with cancer not easily acquired elsewhere: as previously indicated, contact with patients within the health service is too brief to allow for the systematic coverage of patients' concerns at all stages of their illness career. Cancer self-help groups such as CALL are accessible to patients and relatives at all times, including, in the case of CALL's telephone help, the evenings and weekends. Because of this accessibility, CALL is in a position constantly to update itself on what is currently concerning people with cancer and those around them.

The very fact that people under stress are prepared to telephone complete strangers rather than, or as well as, people in the health service with whom they have already been in contact, indicates a need to re-examine what it is necessary to provide to cancer patients and their families, at all stages of the illness. Groups such as CALL are well placed to broaden the agenda of issues relevant to those coping with cancer, and their contribution in the future could be much enhanced if formal systems of communication with health service practitioners were established, whereby information on these issues could be passed on to those responsible for the provision of current services.

References

Brown, T., and Griffiths, P. (1986) 'Cancer Self Help Groups: an Inside View', *British Medical Journal*, **292**, 1503–1504.

Clement-Jones, V. (1985) 'Cancer and Beyond: the Formation of BACUP , *British Medical Journal*, **291**, 1021–1023.

Davison, R. L. (1984) *Knowledge and Opinion about Cancer in Bury, Lancashire, 1980.* Manchester Regional Committee for Cancer Education.

Eardley, A. (1986) 'Patients' Views of Radiotherapy' in Hegarty J. R., and DeCann R. W. (eds.). *Psychology in Radiography.* Change Publication, Stoke-on-Trent.

Eardley, A., and Brown, T. (1985) 'Cancer Line', *Nursing Mirror*, **160**(4) 16–17.

Eardley, A., George, W. D., Davis, F., Schofield, P. F., Wilson, M. C., Wakefield, J., Sellwood, R. A. (1976) 'Colostomy: the Consequences of Surgery', *Clinical Oncology*, **2**, 277–283.

Feldman, F. L. (1978) *Work and Cancer Health Histories: a Study of the Experiences of Recovered Blue Collar Workers: Findings and Implications.* American Cancer Society, New York.

Fobair, P., Hoppe, R. T., Bloom, J., Cox, R., Varghese, A., Spiegel, D. (1986) 'Psychosocial Problems among Survivors of Hodgkin's Disease', *Journal of Clinical Oncology*, **4**, 805–814.

Follick, M. J., Smith, T. W., and Turk, D. C. (1984) 'Psychosocial Adjustment following Ostomy', *Health Psychology*, **3**, 505–517.

Hinton, J. (1973) 'Bearing Cancer', *British Journal of Medical Psychology*, **46**, 105–113.

Houlton, E. A. (1987) 'Cancer—The Challenge to Primary Health Care'. *Journal of the Royal Society of Health*, **4**, 151–154.

Knopf, A. (1976) 'Changes in Women's Opinions about Cancer', *Social Science and Medicine*, **10**, 191–195.

Lock, S. (1986) 'Self Help Groups: the Fourth Estate in Medicine?' *British Medical Journal*, **293**, 1596–1600.

Maguire, G. P., Lee, E. G., Bevington, D. J., Küchemann, C. S., Crabtree, R. J.,

Cornell, C. E. (1978) 'Psychiatric Problems in the First Year after Mastectomy'. *British Medical Journal*, i, 963–965.

Peters-Golden, H. (1982) 'Breast Cancer: Varied Perceptions of Social Support in the Illness Experience', *Social Science and Medicine*, 16, 483–491.

Rieker, P. P., Edbril, S. D., and Garnick, M. B. (1985) 'Curative Testis Cancer Therapy: Psychosocial Sequelae', *Journal of Clinical Oncology*, 3, 1117–1126.

Sontag, S. (1979) *Illness as Metaphor*. Allen Lane, London.

Wortman, C. B., and Dunkel-Schetter, C. (1979) 'Interpersonal Relationships and Cancer: a Theoretical Analysis', *Journal of Social Issues*, 35, 120–155.

Changing Ideas in Health Care
Edited by D. Seedhouse and A. Cribb
© 1989 John Wiley & Sons Ltd

Chapter Four
The Care-by-Parent Scheme: An Innovation in the Hospital Care of Child Patients

JEAN CLEARY
Institute of Health Care Studies
University College of Swansea
UK

Background

The publication of the Platt Report on the Welfare of Children in Hospital in 1959, and the adoption of its recommendations by the Ministry of Health, marked a watershed in the care of children in hospital in Britain. In the period before, visiting children in hospital was strictly limited, generally to a few hours a week, or sometimes totally prohibited (Cleary, 1986). Mothers were permitted to stay with breastfed babies, and permission was granted for both parents to stay with critically ill children. With these exceptions the common belief was that visitors would get in the way of the work and introduce infection to the wards. And since the children always cried at the end of visiting it seemed obvious that it was an upsetting experience that would hinder recovery.

There had been pioneers who contested this accepted wisdom. The best known of these were the paediatricians J. C. Spence and Dermod MacCarthy, who encouraged 'mothering-in', and Agnes Hunt, the matron of the Oswestry orthopaedic hospital, who believed in unrestricted visiting. James Nicoll of Glasgow was another dissident. He wrote (in the *British Medical Journal*, 1909) 'that suckling and young infants should remain with their mothers after operation . . . Even when the child is "bottlefed", separation from the mother is often harmful.'

Observations of the effects of separation on young children during the Second World War began to change thinking. The work of Bowlby (1952) and the Robertsons (e.g. Robertson 1958) (particularly their films) was taken to be conclusive by many. As Martin Richards (1981) says:

> What is not in doubt was that children were very often upset while in hospital and cried for their parents and frequently showed behavioural disturbances after

> they had returned home. Many parents found that the enforced separation was
> very painful . . . Changes only began on any scale when it was argued that the
> separation . . . could have long term psychological consequences for the children.

Obvious unhappiness was insufficient to provoke a change in policy. Indeed, post-discharge behaviour problems were sometimes attributed to the child being spoilt in hospital. Parents who regarded the separation as an ordeal comforted themselves with the notion that the episode was 'character building'.

Once the idea that separation from the mother and other family members (Hall and Stacey, 1979) was harmful was embodied in policy, practice began to change in Western Europe and North America. But there were varying degrees of enthusiasm in different countries and areas (Stenbak, 1986) and among the specialities that treat child patients (Thornes, 1983). Uniform acceptance of unrestricted visiting has not yet occurred, even in Britain. And where it has been introduced the situation is not always harmonious. One mother in the present study stated that when, in another hospital, she suggested that it might help the staff if she came in with her retarded son, the consultant exclaimed 'Now I've heard everything'. There, and in many hospitals, the presence of parents was tolerated but they were seldom given a role to play— other than to play with the children. The phrase 'the captive mother' was coined by one paediatrician (Meadow, 1969) to describe the common experience of resident mothers. Another mother of a case study child gave an account of her frustration when she was a resident parent elsewhere. She was expected 'just to be company', rather than take any part in her daughter's care. This meant that she had to watch while the child was being bathed or fed by unfamiliar hands.

Recognition of the social and psychological needs of children in hospital also resulted in the employment of more specialised staff to provide for them. These staff included play leaders, play therapists and surrogate parents (usually volunteers). There has also been increased educational provision within hospitals and the establishment of 'child life programs'. However, in some cases it has seemed that the semi-professional parent whose responsibility is to the hospital is seen as the best solution to the problem of the sick child 'lying isolated in his crib' (Fineberg and Jones, 1960). This option has been preferred over the alternative of encouraging unrestricted visiting.

This professionalisation was a feature of care in the United States. But during the late 1960s a new movement began in America designed to return the care of at least some children to their parents. The idea was proposed as early as 1961 by the Indianapolis paediatrician Morris Green, but the first care-by-parent unit was set up in Lexington, Kentucky, in 1966 (Lerner, Haley, Hall and McVarish, 1972). The Indianapolis project was set up in 1971 (Green and Green, 1977). Others have been established in various parts of the USA and in Canada during the 1970s and 1980s. The aims of these units are twofold. First, where feasible to allow the child's natural caregivers to nurse the child in hospital and to take the responsibility for that child as they would at home. And second, to reduce the cost of hospitalisation by cutting down on the use of professional staff time.

The Cardiff Scheme

The Paediatric Unit in the University Hospital of Wales was opened in 1972. It has always practised a policy of unrestricted visiting for parents and allowed liberal access to other family members, including children. It has always been possible for one adult to 'live in' with the child. When parents are present they are expected to carry out all the normal personal care and feeding unless there are clinical contra-indications, and to give oral medications. Some parents are also taught to carry out more skilled nursing procedures—those that must be done at home after discharge. Among these are naso-gastric feeding (including passing the tube), tracheostomy care and parenteral feeding. When the setting up of a care-by-parent scheme was suggested, the senior nursing staff regarded it as the next logical step in increasing the involvement of parents in the lives of children in hospital. It was felt that the initiative would extend the range of parents who might take on the nursing care of their children in hospital, and give them the responsibility for care that they have at home, while maintaining supervision.

The North American units generally have separate premises and separate staff. The Cardiff scheme had neither of these, nor did it have any separate funding. Instead, it had to work within the existing establishment and budget of the paediatric unit, as an option within the ordinary ward. Two of the three paediatric wards were suitable because one consisted largely, and the other entirely, of separate cubicles. The latter also already had a parents' lounge, kitchen and bathroom, as well as a washing-machine that the parents could use. It was agreed that the scheme would begin operation at the beginning of May 1984. The Leverhulme Trust funded the writer and a team of observers to carry out a study of the scheme, and to observe other aspects of the lives of children in hospital.

It is clear that not all children can be nursed in a care-by-parent setting. For example the desperately ill are not a suitable category. Guidelines were drawn up for the selection of suitable children. These were:

1. Children who need medical supervision but little skilled nursing care—perhaps those admitted for diagnostic tests or during the later stages of an admission.
2. Children with long-term conditions whose parents will have to learn specific techniques so that the children can go and continue to minimise the effects of the condition. Examples of this category include those children with congenital abnormalities or diabetes.
3. Children whose parents are considered to be in need of more general health education, in diet, hygiene or childrearing practices, in order to improve the health status or prospects of one child or the whole family. One example would be if there were feeding problems or repeated minor infections.

In practice most patients fall into at least one of these categories during some part of their admission. However, the great majority of those in the scheme were in the first two groups rather than the third. The overriding prerequisite was a resident parent, willing and able to take on the tasks and the responsibility.

A leaflet describing the scheme was prepared for parents and an induction procedure agreed. A badge was devised by which the cubicles where the care-by-parent scheme (CBP) was operating could be identified. A smaller version was provided for the CBP nurse. The original was a red teddy bear, but later a panda was adopted, for ease of reproduction in black and white.

The Research Project

Seven women, all with a background in teaching or nursing, were trained as observers by the author, who also acted as an observer. Two main types of non-participant observation were used. One type was 'activity sampling' where a 'snapshot' of what was going on throughout the two wards was taken at 20-minute intervals during the day. The other method was to observe up to three individual children continuously for five minutes in each hour, to provide case studies (23 in the CBP scheme, 21 before it was set up). Precoded sheets were used for both types of observation. The day was defined as lasting from 6.15 a.m. to 11.30 p.m. approximately.

Each observer also kept a diary of events between observations to amplify what was contained in the coded sheets. All the data were supplemented by a questionnaire to nurses before the scheme began operation, and a post-discharge structured interview with the parents of case study children (21 CBP and 17 others). There were also many informal discussions with parents and staff throughout the project.

Joining the Scheme

When a child was thought suitable for the care-by-parent scheme and had a resident parent,* the parent was approached by a senior registrar or ward sister who told her something about the scheme and asked if she would consider joining it. The parents' questions were answered, they were given the leaflet to read, and time to think about and discuss the idea. If the parent decided to take part, she was introduced to the CBP nurse and the learning process began.

On each shift one nurse was chosen as CBP nurse. The nurse needed to be experienced in paediatric nursing and in communicating with parents, and needed to have sufficient maturity to teach and support them. Sometimes the senior sister could take on the job and sometimes, because of staffing difficulties or the presence of seriously ill children, it was necessary to involve a junior nurse. No special training was given, so natural aptitude was important.

The first procedures taught were the taking and charting of the routine observations of temperature, pulse and respiration. Obviously this cannot all be done at once and the principle was that the parent should take over full

---

*The term 'parent' has been used throughout. It refers more often to mothers, but some fathers undertook the care or shared it with their wives. One grandmother was the carer during the observation period. Since the majority were women the pronoun 'she' is used.

responsibility for one of them (or any other procedures) only when she felt confident and the CBP nurse considered her competent. Temperature taking was usually the easiest, although taking the rectal temperature of babies sometimes caused anxiety. Many parents, and even some nurses, find it difficult to take a baby's pulse. Generally the process began with the nurse taking the temperature, showing the parent how it was done, how to read the result and then how to enter it on the chart. The next stage was for the nurse to take the temperature of the child, checking the parent's reading and charting it, followed by the parent doing it under supervision until finally taking over.

In general the project progressed smoothly, although there could be initial difficulties (Sainsbury, Gray, Cleary, Davies and Rowlandson, 1986) and occasional confusions. The most common reason for a parent not assuming responsibility was the early discharge of the child. The mean length of stay for CBP patients, who were mainly babies, was six days, but half of them stayed three days or less. This does not allow much time for learning. However, since temperature was taken at four-hourly intervals or less, there were several opportunities on each day. In the very early days, as a part of the educational process, both mother and CBP nurse felt the pulse for the regulation period. But eventually it was recognised that the mother did not know she was supposed to be counting. Some nurses found it difficult to comprehend that a parent might know so little, perhaps less than the nurse herself had known before she began her training. This particular problem was easily solved, by counting aloud in the early stages of learning the technique.

What each parent learned to do was dependent on the needs of her own child and the time available—one child was brought into the scheme and was adopted for case study, only to be discharged two hours later, without any real opportunity for participation.

Tasks which were undertaken by parents included:

    taking temperature,
    checking pulse,
    checking respiration,
    watching infusions,
    giving oral medications by syringe,
    measuring fluid intake,
    urine collection,
    stool collection,
    naso-gastric feeds,
    passing naso-gastric tube,
    naso-pharyngeal suction,
    chest percussion and postural drainage,
    nebuliser treatment,
    using apnoea alarm,
    parenteral nutrition,
    tracheostomy care,
    stoma care.
    (See the glossary at the end of this chapter for an explanation of terms used.)

When the task had been carried out, the parent recorded it in the notes. The diaries and data sheets include the following examples:

1. Mother shakes down thermometer, takes temperature, pulse. Checks with staff, records.
2. Sister explains mechanics of IVI equipment, including flow of liquid. Mother listens attentively, checks notes, converses with sister.
3. Temperature has just been taken. Checks drip, sees that it is nearly empty. Fetches SEN, who checks—shows mother how to check burette and top it up.
4. Father looks at notes and makes entry . . . Mother and father talk about nursing care, father explaining something to mother. He passes notes to mother. They discuss how much fluid going through drip.
5. Sister shows mother how to attach urine collection bag.
6. Mother sucks out tracheostomy, stopping to change inner tube. Baby unhappy towards end of procedure.

Effects on the Children

Most of the children in the CBP scheme were patients in what was primarily an infants' ward. Their average age was 34 weeks (range 3–95 weeks). During the 'activity sampling' it was possible to compare the lives of three groups of children: those without a resident parent (NR), those with a resident parent (RP) and those in the CBP scheme (CBP) (Cleary, Gray, Hall, Rowlandson, Sainsbury and Davies, 1986). The ward consisted of 14 cubicles. Using a folding bed, the parent shared the cubicle with the child.

The most striking variations were between those with a resident parent (RP or CBP) and those without (NR). Those without spent more than two-thirds of the observed day alone, while for those with it was a little more than a quarter. These proportions include sleep, but when those for 'observed alone and awake' (a condition likely to be distressing for a sick infant in a strange place) are examined, there are significant differences between the three (see Table 1). Resident parents who were not in the scheme, perhaps because their involvement in care was minor or because they had less confidence in their ability to do anything valuable, were more likely to be absent.

Table 1

Group	Alone and awake (percentage of observations)
NR	19.8
RP	9.4
CBP	3.4
No. of direct observations = 4225	

Direct observations = the number of observation rounds × children present and visible.

Children 'in company' may be with parents, other family members, friends, or with members of the nursing or medical staff or other health care professionals. The NR children had the majority of their contacts with nurses (66 per cent). This means that the children contacted quite a large number of individuals over a few days. They had more contacts with qualified nurses and with student nurses than they did with their mothers. Mothers are the most frequent contacts for both the other groups, but RP children see much less of their fathers and other members of their families. The CBP children as a group had more than a quarter of their contacts with their fathers, who might have been the parent-carer, sharing care with the mother, or visiting.

RP and CBP children had 8 and 4 per cent respectively of their contact with staff alone. The proportion of contacts with family and friends for the three groups were NR 27 per cent; RP 75 per cent; CBP 83 per cent. The remaining class of contacts were with both staff and family, which included occasions when nursing or other professional care was being carried out. This time is also particularly important for the exchange of information and teaching. The figures for the three groups are NR 7 per cent; RP 17 per cent; CBP 13 per cent.

With very young children the amount of crying might be considered to be an indicator of distress or some unmet need. The figures in Table 2 support the idea that the CBP child will be the least unhappy and his or her needs will be attended to most quickly.

Those without a resident parent cried more than the others and on half the occasions they were alone. Total crying and the proportion alone is reduced for the children with a resident parent and both are less again for those in the CBP scheme.

Evaluation

The simple distress of the child in hospital has not in the past been considered sufficient reason for changing hospital practice, and there has been no opportunity to carry out a long-term follow-up to assess the effects of this innovation in care. However, the immediate effects on the CBP case study

Table 2 Amount of time spent crying

	Crying (percentage of observations made when child was awake)		
	NR	RP	CBP
Crying alone	11	4	2
Crying in company	11	13	11
Total crying	21	18	13
Total number of observations while awake	1211	338	518

Reproduced by permission of *Archives of Disease in Childhood.*

children were reported by parents in the post-discharge interview and can be compared, to a certain extent, with a group who were case study children before the scheme began operation. These children were selected because their medical condition would have been appropriate for care-by-parent, had it existed at the time. Some had resident parents and some did not. The group included children with a higher average age (2 years 9 months). In this interview, based on a questionnaire (see Appendix), parents were asked about the child's behaviour when he or she went home. Did they, in the parent's estimation, return to normal straightaway? Did they show improvement or problems in mood, feeding, sleeping and other aspects of behaviour?

The interviews were carried out two to four weeks after discharge, when parents of 19 CBP children (two gave no opinion) and 17 from the earlier phase, gave answers which may be summarized as follows:

1. CBP children
   - nine back to normal straightaway,
   - ten showed some behavioural disturbance, two considered to be 'still ill', five disturbed for less than one week, three still showing some disturbance.

2. Pre-CBP children
   - seven back to normal straightaway (four RP) (including three 'veterans' over five years old)
   - eight showed, or still showing, some behavioural disturbance (five RP)
   - two too young or too unresponsive to distinguish the effects of hospitalisation (two RP).

'Veteran' means a child who has a chronic condition (two of these were diabetics) and who has had many admissions, probably well into double figures. 'Veterans' were accustomed to both the ward and the treatment they would receive and, although they were not always happy, they were relatively untroubled by the experience.

The main problems mentioned by the CBP parents were that the children were being very clinging, and that there were feeding and sleeping difficulties. Only two mentioned 'bad temper'. Among the pre-CBP children (both RP and NR) factors such as difficult behaviour, aggressiveness, 'being spiteful', 'being bad tempered and disobedient' were mentioned of six of the eight considered to have been disturbed by their experience. There was considerable variation among the members of the three groups, but the results suggest that those who were in the CBP scheme were less disturbed, or disturbed for a shorter period. (Obviously, the results of such a small study cannot be considered conclusive.)

The Experience of the Parent-Carers

It is highly significant that nearly all the parents were quite clear that if their child were readmitted they would want to be in a CBP scheme again. The one grandmother who took part felt that it was too much responsibility at times, but would do it again. One father who shared care with his wife did not think that he would have been able to take it on by himself. The only real exception was a very young single mother who was dissatisfied with the diagnosis of her son's condition; she felt that the responsibility should be with the nurse. However, she said that she would 'like to do as much as possible—if he cried I would know I had hurt him—nobody else'.

Some felt they were 'tied' to the ward, which is a reflection of the conscientiousness with which they carried out their tasks. Some parents scarcely left the ward. Snacks and drinks could be made in the parents' kitchen, but main meals were generally taken in the staff cafeteria. This was a long way from the Paediatric Unit. Consequently most were reluctant to be away as long as it would take to go, eat and come back unless they were sure that the child was sound asleep or the other parent was there. Five had their meals brought in to them, two said they 'couldn't eat anyway' and the sharing father mentioned above, 'just went without'.

Most of them felt that their confidence in dealing with illness in general had increased, except for two who had not been in the scheme long enough to learn much and those who were already skilled (two with nursing training and one couple who were doing a great deal at home before this admission). Comments made to Sainsbury et al. (1986) suggest that parents regard the main benefit to the child to be living with familiar people who are trusted, even when they were doing unfamiliar, even uncomfortable, things. Parents had no other commitments in the ward beyond the care of their own child and could, therefore, give medication or do observations at the most suitable times for that child. From the parents' point of view, the advantages were that they were part of the team and could take an active part in promoting the child's recovery. At a more prosaic level, simply having things to do made the hospital stay less boring and frustrating for the parent (Meadow, 1969). One parent said, 'If you're there you might as well—[I] enjoyed doing as much as I could'.

As reported by an observer, the mother of one 16-month-old girl, admitted for investigations

> was surprised at being asked to join in the CBP scheme, but thought it was a nice idea. It was less boring because she has things to do—she had been taught to take temperatures rectally and the child did not struggle as much as when they do it under the arm. She collects faecal specimens if required, records fluid intake and when wet [i.e. output] which is sometimes done by strict collection and sometimes by weighing nappies. It keeps down the number handling the child and there's always a friendly face around, so she doesn't get upset.

A six-week-old baby who was not gaining weight was also being investigated. Her mother said that she had 'learned how to take temperatures, but not pulse or respiration, because she is so small . . . I liked writing the notes and feeling that I have a right to read them'.

When the senior registrar went canvassing reactions, he reported 'pleasure from all parties, especially at writing medication and urine collection notes'. It seems to have been this aspect of CBP which convinced parents that there was a real change in responsibility, and that they were not just taking part in a cosmetic exercise.

Problems

The complaints which parents voiced mainly concerned the distance to the cafeteria and sleeping in such a busy place, rather than anything specifically to do with the scheme, although some would have welcomed more reassurance from staff.

An American study (Monaghan and Schkade, 1985) suggests that parents in a CBP unit, for handicapped children being taught to walk for the first time, became more anxious than those in conventional care, but 'gave almost unanimously positive responses about their satisfaction with spending greater amounts of time with their children and being given responsibility for their care'.

The biggest problem for those families with more than one child was arranging care for the siblings. Grandmothers were the principle carers, mentioned seven times, and friends were cited three times. Three fathers and two mothers took time off work (one took holiday time).

Being resident in hospital entailed material costs for all the families. These costs included fares or petrol, working time lost, meals in hospital, the need to buy more or newer clothes, and nearly everyone felt compelled to buy presents for the patient. Apart from loss of earnings, expenses were estimated by 16 parents at between £8 and £40. Time off work was variously reckoned to have cost from £20 to £250. The hardest hit was a supply teacher who turned down jobs while resident. A child who is chronically ill and frequently in hospital can be a considerable drain on the family income. One couple had 'got behind with their mortgage' and feared that the time off might cost the husband his job.

The Role of the Nurse

Without the wholehearted support of the nursing staff the CBP scheme could not work. The research study was principally concerned with the effects of the scheme on the children and their parents, not because the effects on the nurses were considered to be less important but because funds for this aspect of the project were not forthcoming.

The role of the nurse with responsibility for the CBP patients is to teach, supervise and support the parents. The initial stage of introducing a mother or father into the scheme requires a great deal of nurse-time—to explain the nature and purpose of a procedure and to teach the techniques for carrying it out and recording it. When the parent is judged competent and confident to carry out the necessary tasks unaided the nurse maintains supervision and continues to offer reassurance. Teaching procedures takes up more of the nurse's time than carrying them out would and teaching may continue for a long time when a child has a chronic condition. For example, the parents of a child with a malabsorption syndrome learned, over many weeks, basic nursing care, then naso-gastric feeding, then the management of infusions and finally parenteral nutrition. If no complex procedures are involved there will be a reduction in the nursing time needed, compared with conventional nursing care, but these children will probably stay a relatively short time in hospital. The American CBP units often exist without any assigned nursing staff, but with the normal flow of work within the Welsh wards, the variation in the numbers in CBP and the demands their conditions make upon the staff, there is no suggestion that staffing could be reduced. Nurses have not voiced any anxiety about losing jobs, but the question has been raised several times by parents.

Teaching parents to carry out the tasks of professionals seemed to arouse little conflict: senior nurses, in particular, are accustomed to instructing their juniors and, though some parents may be more ignorant of nursing matters than a newly recruited nursing auxiliary, the knowledge base of most is probably broadly similar and their motivation in regard to the one child much stronger. In one series of 32 CBP cases, nurses were asked to assess parents' performance (Sainsbury *et al.*, 1986) and they

> considered that the parents performed the tasks satisfactorily in 30 of the 32 cases. In 15 instances they considered that the standards were, in fact, better . . . The nurses believed that their relationships with the parents were in fact better than in the traditional method and enjoyed their teaching and supervisory roles in 30 out of the 32 cases. They found that it was not difficult to teach parents the skills required.

One senior sister said that she felt that conversation between the nurse and the parent was more informative and useful than in the traditional setting. Another felt that discussions with doctors were also more productive.

The main worry expressed before the scheme began operation was that parents would not perceive the significance of changes in the vital signs and that deterioration, which in babies may be very rapid might be unnoticed. Nothing of this nature occurred. In fact, parents seem too conscious of the most minor fluctuations, according to one nurse.

Nurses were called upon to make decisions about parents in the scheme. One mother was removed from it, during the observation period, because she was not felt to be sufficiently conscientious. Staff were also worried about her general style of child management and, if there had been more staff experienced in running CBP, it would have been possible to increase education and supervision. Sometimes a father who was relieving his wife as carer proved less proficient and staff would take over until she returned. It was often necessary to urge the carer, particularly the single mothers, to take a break from the ward and the hospital or to go home for a night, now and then, during a long admission.

The post-discharge questionnaires to parents asked some questions about their relationships with the nurses. Nearly everyone said that they had been sympathetic and patient. There was some feeling that nurses outside the scheme were unsympathetic. Parents' ratings of the teaching varied a good deal more, most regarding it as good and sufficient, but five felt that 'too much was expected too quickly', and three wanted more help with taking the pulse.

There should always have been at least one CBP nurse, identifiable by means of badge, to whom the parents could turn for help and advice, and nine (of 21) said there was no difficulty in finding her or him. Seven, however, did not seem to know that this was what they should be doing and five said the CBP nurse was difficult to find. Two of the last group said that the nurse should always have introduced her or himself and made a point of 'popping in and out'. However, a parent who had experienced no problems described the CBP nurses as doing exactly that. The observations suggest that nurses tended to check on the child and the record keeping when the parents had gone for a break or a meal. But the parents would have welcomed the extra contact and the reassurance that the professionals' approval of their performance would bring.

The greatest potential for conflict existed at night. The night staff, fewer in number and often part-time, had been less involved in setting up the scheme. They sometimes found the presence of parents at different stages of involvement and competence confusing and time-consuming compared with traditional care.

Discussion

Care-by-parent clearly works from the point of view of the children. They spend less time alone, have most of their care and contact from familiar people and cry less. Parents felt that post-hospital disturbance was less. The nursing care given by instructed parents was satisfactory or better in nearly every case, and in only one (of approximately 50 cases) was it felt necessary to withdraw the parent from the scheme. Parents learned to carry out a wide variety of procedures, some of which are very complex and even dangerous if performed incompetently. They liked being in the scheme and would do it again. The satisfaction of having an essential part to play in the nursing care and of having a meaningful occupation outweighed the anxiety that their unfamiliar tasks could induce.

The nurses who did the teaching did not find that parting with their knowledge conflicted with their professional status—teaching some parents some procedures has been part of their function for a long time. It was, however, more time-consuming in the early stages and some parents felt the need for more time. Nurses did not always comprehend the total lack of knowledge of some of their pupils, the need for continuing reinforcement of the teaching, and the need to reassure parents about performance. These variations were bound to occur when 'the designated nurse' had to change from shift to shift. This means that there is little chance of always selecting the person best qualified for the job, when other pressures of nursing work must be taken into account. Those who acted as CBP nurses seldom got the opportunity to build up real expertise.

Despite this reservation, it is clear from the evidence collected about the care-by-parent scheme that it can work, despite the complete absence of specific staffing or extra funding within the normal functioning of the ward. The new option did not disrupt the work of the ward, but sometimes had to give way to the need for skilled hands-on nursing, since the CBP nurse had to be an experienced paediatric nurse. This, coupled with the fact that the scheme operates at ward level, means that the option may not always be offered consistently. To avoid the likelihood of erratic operation, it seems essential that there should be at least one nurse whose sole or principal responsibility is to the CBP scheme.

The Paediatric Unit did possess some facilities for parents, which were minimal in comparison with the pavilions of North America, but sufficient to make the constricted life of a resident parent tolerable.

A hospital which is interested in the care-by-parent idea, and which has the choice, must consider whether to include it in the existing wards, as has been done in Cardiff, or to set up a separate unit. A planned unit would presumably have adequate facilities for the children and their parents, even if it did not rise to the standards of motel accommodation. It would have its own staff, who would not have to face the dilemmas that arose within the ordinary wards. Staff would also be able to develop expertise in their educational and supportive role. A separate unit would, on the other hand, have a fixed number of beds to fill, which might mean turning away suitable children.

When CBP is part of the ordinary ward, the decision to offer participation can be made at any suitable time during the admission, which increases its availability to a wide range of children. Having agreed that CBP is appropriate, entry to the scheme is not dependent on the availability of a bed nor does it require physical removal to another area. Similarly, leaving the scheme or relinquishing participation temporarily can be achieved without upheaval. Breaks for parents during a long stay or a return to traditional nursing care for the period immediately following surgery, for example, are easily arranged.

The prevailing atmosphere of the ward is also of crucial importance. Wards where parents' presence is less than wholly acceptable and where they are not involved in care to any extent, would find it very difficult to incorporate a radical change in the status and function of parents. There, a separate unit would have a greater chance of success.

Whichever route is chosen, whether the inauguration of the care-by-parent scheme as an option within the framework of the ordinary ward or as the system in an area devoted exclusively to care-by-parent, it can be a valuable additional means of lessening the trauma of hospitalisation. Parents learn to provide optimal care for the chronically sick or handicapped child. It also has potential in the field of more general health education since health professionals make contact with a wide variety of families.

References

Bowlby, J. (1952) *Maternal Care and Mental Health*. World Health Organization, Geneva.

Cleary, J. (1986) 'The Child in Hospital and the Re-emergence of the Family', in Cule, J. and Turner, T. (eds.), *Child Care through the Centuries*. STS Publishing, Cardiff.

Cleary, J., Gray, O. P., Hall, D. J., Rowlandson, P. H., Sainsbury, C. P. Q., and Davies, M. M. (1986), 'Parental Involvement in the Lives of Children in Hospital', *Archives of Disease in Childhood*, **61**, 779–787.

Fineberg, H., and Jones, E. (1960) 'Morther Bank in a Children's Hospital', *Journal of the American Medical Association*, **174**, 2153–2154.

Green, M., and Green, J. G. (1977) 'The Parent Care Pavilion', *Child Today* **6**, 5–8.

Hall, D. J., and Stacey, M. (1979) *Beyond Separation*. Routledge, London.

Lerner, M., Haley, J., Hall, D., and McVarish, D. (1972) 'Hospital Care-by-Parent: an Evaluative Look', *Medical Care*, **10**, 430–436.

Meadow, S. (1969) 'The Captive Mother', *Archives of Disease in Childhood*, **44**, 362–367.

Monaghan, G., and Schkade, J. (1985) 'Comparing Care by Parent and Traditional Nursing Units', *Pediatric Nursing*, **11**, 463–468.

Richards, M. P. M. (1981) 'Aspects of Development in Contemporary Society', in Chester, R. Diggory, P. and Sutherland, M. (eds.), *Changing Patterns of Childbearing and Child Rearing*. Academic Press, London.

Robertson, J. (1958) *The Young Child in Hospital*. Tavistock, London.

Sainsbury, C. P. Q., Gray, O. P., Cleary, J., Davies, M. M., and Rowlandson, P.H. (1986) 'Care by Parents of their Children in Hospital', *Archives of Disease in Childhood*, **61**, 612–615.

Stenbak, E. (1986) *Care of Children in Hospital*. World Health Organisation, Regional Office for Europe, Copenhagen.

Thornes, R. (1983) 'Parental Access and Family Facilities in Children's Wards in England', *British Medical Journal*, **287**, 190–192.

Glossary

Watching infusions When nutrients or medication are introduced directly into the blood stream, 'being on a drip', the quantity of liquid in the bag or bottle, the rate of flow and the condition of the point of entry must all be monitored.

Oral medication by syringe Liquid medicine is squirted into the baby's mouth from a syringe without a needle.

Naso-gastric feeding, 'tube feeding' Extra liquids and food needed by babies and small children may be given directly through a tube passed into the nose, down the gullet and into the stomach.

Naso-pharyngeal suction A method of clearing fluid from the air passages.

Chest percussion and postural drainage, 'tilt and tap' The patient lies with head lower than feet, and the chest and back are tapped vigorously, in order to help expel excessive secretions from the lungs; used several times a day in cystic fibrosis.

Nebuliser treatment Medicated liquid reduced to a very fine spray is inhaled through a mask, in order to loosen lung secretions; often used before chest percussion.

Apnoea alarm Device set up in a baby's cot, which sounds when the baby stops breathing.

Parenteral nutrition or intravenous feeding When prolonged, parents learned the complete management of infusions.

Tracheostomy care When an artificial airway has been constructed, with a tube into the windpipe, the tube must be kept clear of secretions and the inner tube changed when necessary.

Stoma care An artificial opening from the intestine through the abdominal wall (colostomy or ileostomy) has been constructed, through which faecal matter is discharged into a bag. The bags must be attached securely, changed regularly.

Appendix

INSTITUTE OF HEALTH CARE STUDIES
UNIVERSITY COLLEGE SWANSEA

POST HOSPITAL QUESTIONNAIRE

1. Name

4. Hospital No.

2. Date of birth

5. Age at admission

3. Address

6. House, flat, part, shared accommodation

7. Household composition

8. Length of stay

9. Continuous, leave, readmission

10. Care-by-parent—how long?

11.   Has s/he been in hospital before?

12.   Admission planned/emergency
route—parent, GP-R, GP-S, OP, ward

13.   Were you expecting admission?

14.   How ill was s/he on admission?

15.   What were the symptoms?

16.   Did you intend to stay anyway?

17.   Who stayed? M, F, both, alternating, mainly M
Specify any other

18.   Other children

19.   How have you managed?

20.   Did being in hospital cause extra expense?

Fares/petrol	Meals in hospital
New clothing	Care for other children
Presents	Time off work Mother
Other	Father

21.   Could you estimate the total cost?

22.   Are you working?
Looking for work?

23.   Is there a male breadwinner in the family?
What is his job?
Is he employed at the moment?
If not, how long?

Baby

24.   Do you think that . . . . was old enough to notice anything different
about being in hospital?

25.   Is s/he normally: happy/miserable/wants attention
sleeps well/badly
feeds well/badly

26.   How did s/he behave in hospital?

27.   At home again — back to normal straightaway?

problems or	feeding
improvements	sleeping
	clinging
	crying more

more contented
livelier

not really recovered yet

Child

30. Do you think that . . . . was old enough to
    notice the difference
    at first too ill to care
    upset by it
    contented while M or F, other there
    settled down quickly

31. Is . . . . normally
    happy/miserable
    quiet/active
    adventurous/stays close

32. Does s/he
    eat well/badly
    sleep well/badly

33. How did s/he behave in hospital?

34. After going home, back to normal?
    straightaway, soon, not yet?
    problems or improvements?   feeding
                                                sleeping
                                                clinging
                                                more independent
                                                bad tempered
                                                better tempered
                                                aggressive

35. Was it possible to explain anything?

36. Have you talked about it since going home?

Care-by-Parent Nursing

37. Which of these did
    you do in hospital
    or do at home?

    i.   take temperature
    ii.   respiration
    iii.   pulse
    iv.   fluid intake
    v.   urine collection
    vi.   medication oral
    vii. nasogastric feed
    viii.   medication
    ix.   pass tube
    x.   drip check
              change bag
    xi.   oxygen tent
                  mask
    xii. mist tent
    xiii. nebuliser
    xiv   chest suction
    xv.   stoma care
    xvi. physiotherapy
    xvii. other

HOSPITAL				HOME
Nurses	Attempt	Did	Charted	B/A

38. Did you accompany to X-ray or operating theatre?

39. Did s/he have   blood tests?
                     biopsy?
                     injections?
                     other?

Parents' opinions of care-by-parent

40. Good idea, would do again?
    too much of a tie?
    too much responsibility

41. How did you arrange your own breaks?

42. What did you think of the facilities for parents' meals, sleeping, etc?

43. How soon was care-by-parent mentioned to you?

44. Who by?

45. How long did it take you to make up your mind?

46. Do you think that the system was explained well beforehand?

47. Did you find the booklet adequate?

48. Were there problems?   finding the right nurse
                              getting information

49. Did you ever find that a nurse had done something, e.g. temperature, that you were going to do, without checking with you first?

50. Was TPR explained well, too much expected too quickly?

51. Were the nurses who explained sympathetic, patient?

52. How many were involved in teaching you?

53. Did you find the other mothers friendly?

54. Did they help with information about things on the ward
                                              in the hospital

55. Did they show you how to do things, e.g. temperature, or help you with them?

56. Do you feel that your confidence in dealing with illness has increased?

57. Would you take temperatures, etc. at home?

58. Do you think that you could learn other things, e.g. nasogastric tube, injections?

Part II
Changing Communities

Introduction to Part II

Just as medicine is changing as a result of taking the themes of holism, equality and autonomy seriously, so is work to improve community health. The five projects included in this section all seek to improve the lives of communities by fostering the participation of community members. In part this can be seen as spreading the responsibility previously shouldered by health professionals, but what is more important is that it involves enabling people to identify and address their own needs.

Alex Scott-Samuel reflects on the history of the Speke Neighbourhood Health Group, which he sees as a forerunner of what has come to be called the 'new public health movement'. John Ashton describes the WHO Healthy Cities project, as it applies to Merseyside, as one manifestation of this popular crusade. There are a number of reasons why these authors have come to speak of a 'new wave' or a renaissance in public health promotion. First, the proportionate increase of non-infectious diseases and life problems that require cultural and lifestyle changes, and hence community interventions. Second, there has been a reassessment, and re-learning, of the strengths and successes of the traditional public health role, as compared with medical and surgical interventions. Third, the growth of grass-roots self-help initiatives over recent years that has coincided with the development of new holistic models of health promotion, many of which have been popularised and disseminated by the WHO 'health for all by the year 2000' strategy. In brief, these models call for an expansion of the conventional health education role so as to include personal empowerment and social policy as well as health information.

The Speke group that Scott-Samuel discusses was set up to identify the needs of a small, economically depressed, neighbourhood in Liverpool, to act as a forum for the exchange of information, and as a lobby to push for specific changes. The representatives of the group were drawn from a range of professional and voluntary agencies with an interest in Speke. This approach has many advantages over the 'top-down' approach to health promotion. Individual communities just like individual people, have diverse sets of needs and resources that cannot be fully accommodated by any general policy.

Another advantage of the local approach to health is that the interdependence of health and social conditions ceases to be a theoretical abstraction because it is manifest in the immediate circumstances. Scott-Samuel observes that one of the most satisfying aspects of the group's functioning was the clarity with which people who worked away from the health arena understood, 'that poor nutrition, poverty, lack of education, social isolation or unemployment prevent people living healthy lives'. Yet despite these advantages, this kind of initiative often comes to be seen as a political challenge to the local authority and to the health authority model of health care.

One method of reducing political resistance is to change the perception of public health issues so that they come to be seen not as a specialist hobby horse, but as common property. This is one of the objectives of the WHO Healthy Cities Project that Ashton describes. It can only come about if people begin to think about health in a different way: 'The ultimate plan is that a comprehensive approach to health promotion should incorporate all aspects of city life including architecture, transport and recreation as well as employment, housing, education and medical care'.

Ashton, echoing the rhetoric of the WHO, sees 'the formulation of concepts' and 'the dissemination of ideas' as major elements of the project. Basic to these ideas is the interpretation of health as a flourishing way of life rather than a relatively disease-free condition, and the belief that promoting health is the business of every individual and every sector of society. Thus, health professionals are not only called upon to adapt their own practices but to create a healthy physical and cultural environment through any means open to them.

Disseminating these and related ideas is laying the foundations for a broader-based approach to health care. The long-term success of the project will depend upon the extent to which it is possible to translate the concepts and models developed by the WHO into practical work, and in the latter part of his chapter Ashton cites recent initiatives in Merseyside to illustrate the basis for future developments.

Heartbeat Wales, the project discussed by John Catford and Richard Parish, is a national health promotion campaign that is informed by many of the same models as the two Merseyside initiatives. The ultimate medical objective is to reduce the level of cardiovascular disease in Wales, and, among other things, this depends on achieving success with regard to the conventional health education targets of changing smoking, eating and exercise behaviour. However, the project has adopted a very broad-ranging strategy that aims to build upon existing networks and activities as well as developing new ones, and to work in (as well as across) many sectors of society.

The authors set out the theoretical sources of their methods. These include social marketing techniques which use the power of the mass media to stimulate or reinforce action at the individual and community levels. They also discuss the health promotion process, arguing that 'those who have changed their lifestyles should be encouraged to move from the role of recipient to that of provider, from audience to actor'. This two-way relationship between the personal and the population approaches is central to health promotion. It is not sufficient solely to aim to develop the personal skills and confidence of individuals, or solely to aim to remove social or structural obstacles to welfare. Neither task can be particularly successful without the other.

The last two chapters in Part II relate to community services. Karen Newbigging and Tony Cadman describe 'Powell St', a community mental health service, and Sally Cawley and her fellow workers describe the role of the North Manchester Women's Health Team. Both of these schemes were planned, and are run, in conjunction with the local community in order to identify and respond to needs, and to provide a service by developing and mobilising community resources. These projects also share an anti-discrimination philosophy, which means that they have to target the community as a whole in order to challenge perceptions and institutional constraints, as well as working with particular individuals who seek advice or support.

The Powell Street team outline the thorough planning process that shaped their subsequent work, planning that was informed by carefully articulated values and not, as so often, by convention or by available resources. The universal and basic needs for recognition and autonomy form the heart of these values, so that caring for those with mental health problems is not reduced to treating disorders but aims to promote a satisfying and fulfilling life.

Services such as this also have a profoundly important role in educating the general population about mental health. After all, who could claim to be immune to mental health problems? In helping to remove the stigma associated with mental ill-health they are attacking one of the greatest obstacles to the achievement of human welfare, because often it is only stigma that stands in the way of our finding and sharing constructive steps towards more autonomy and fulfilment.

The Powell Street project is important because it shows the level of planning and the amount of care essential to a real community approach to mental health, at a time when it is sometimes claimed that community care is a less demanding option.

The women's health movement grew out of the mismatch between women's needs and their experiences of health care and it has produced much of the theoretical and political critique of medicalisation, paternalism and reductionism. The North Manchester Women's Health Team's aim is to apply the philosophies of the womens health movement to preventive health care. In practice this means responding to the demands of women by building resources, providing information and support, organising group work and special events in an effort to develop a co-ordinated approach to women's health, and establishing it in the mainstream of service provision. The team is based in a small house which also serves as a drop-in centre. As with Powell Street, every effort is made to make the service accessible. Both project teams stress that the actual physical space they occupy is homely and welcoming, and the importance of this can be seen from another of the shared themes: the widespread suffering caused by women facing isolation, or the loss or absence of a valued role. Cawley notes that, 'Physical and emotional isolation are two of the most powerful and insidious determinants of women's ill-health'. By bringing individuals together for mutual support, health workers are not only restoring their confidence and quality of life, but they are also establishing links that form the beginning of new community feelings, and of future participation.

Changing Ideas in Health Care
Edited by D. Seedhouse and A. Cribb
© 1989 John Wiley & Sons Ltd

Chapter Five
The New Public Health: Speke Neighbourhood Health Group

ALEX SCOTT-SAMUEL
Consultant in Public Health
Liverpool Health Authority
Liverpool
UK

Speke is the first area in the country to have a Neighbourhood Health Group. This Group was set up jointly by the Liverpool Health Authority and City Council so that the views of the many different kinds of local health, social and community workers and residents of the area could be taken into account. The Group has been established for six months and meets in Speke on a two-monthly basis. While it is chaired by Dr Alex Scott-Samuel of Liverpool Health Authority the remainder of the 30 members work in, or have responsibilities covering Speke; they include representatives from school and child health, community nursing, the Community Health Council, environmental health, social work, probation, police, education, DHSS, housing and voluntary and community organisations including Speke Together, Speke Enterprise Centre, the Citizens' Advice Bureau, Age Concern and Crescent 73 Mental Health Association.

People tend to think of health only in relation to family doctors and hospitals, and members of the Group have been keen to share their experience and knowledge about health-related issues and to have a say in influencing the policies of the Health and Local Authorities which affect the health of people in Speke. Topics covered so far by the Group have included health aspects of housing, environmental health and unemployment. The Group hopes to sponsor a survey of primary care needs in the Speke area.

(Speke Press, 1982)

Introduction

This chapter describes the beginnings, existence and premature end of the Speke Neighbourhood Health Group, and places it in its context as a forerunner of the 'new public health movement' that is now coming into its own in the second half of the 1980s.

Beginnings

In 1976–1977 six Neighbourhood Health Workers were appointed as part of the first initiative in community development health work in the UK. Julia Hallam was appointed in Liverpool. The other posts were in London, Belfast, Derry, Sheffield and Milton Keynes. Only one of the six projects survived beyond the one-year period for which funding was made available by 'Alternative Society' (later the 'Foundation for Alternatives'), but the initiative was important in establishing the principle of non-professional neighbourhood health promotion work in the UK. The interdependence of health and social conditions, especially in areas of poverty and deprivation, and the consequent need for local, community-based health action were established elements of health programmes 'exported' by Britain to Third World countries, and had also featured in the 1960s 'War on Poverty' in the USA. However, prior to 1976 no such projects existed in the UK.

During the following decade, the number of projects in this field was to increase from the initial six to 12,000 (Watt, 1986) and the resulting community health movement has been a major force in the renaissance of public health that is now firmly established in (mainly urban) local authorities and communities around the UK. Another important contribution was that of the Unit for the Study of Health Policy (USHP) at Guy's Hospital Medical School in London. In a series of publications in the decade following the 1974 National Health Service (NHS) reorganisation, the unit effectively redefined the basis of the new specialism of community medicine. There was a move away from the faceless bureaucracy of hospital managers. Instead, the unit encouraged the advent of accountable public health advocates, who are not afraid of political conflict or controversy if this is necessary to protect or promote the health of the people.

While much still remains to be done before the unit's ideas become the universal reality, some have already borne fruit—most notably the Health Promotion Teams (HPTs) first described in 'Rethinking Community Medicine' (USHP, 1979). Many, if not most, district health authorities now have Health Promotion Teams—though these are usually a lot more parochial and less concerned with non-NHS health issues than were the teams envisaged by the USHP:

> At the local level the work would involve watch-dog activities, such as scrutinising public and private organisations in the locality and bringing any abnormalities or 'bad' practices (from the point of view of health) into public view. In pursuance of this objective, local groups could be brought together to enable joint consideration of policies and practices which would promote health. Thus reciprocal relationships would be developed with the local media, public meetings held, talks given and so on. Groups involved might include trade union and employer representatives, Health and Safety staff, neighbourhood councils, housing assocations, law centres and charities. Local HPTs would continuously analyse and publicise the local health effects of new and old public policies— whether the policies were local, national or otherwise. For example, they would scrutinise local authority policy in such relevant areas as environmental health, transport, recreation and housing.

(USHP, 1979, p.82)

In 1981, in Liverpool, it seemed to be time to translate these ideas into reality. I developed the idea of a Neighbourhood Health Group, which was to combine campaigning on issues of public policy with practical organising in the local community. It seemed important to root it in the official NHS structure, so that it would have some chance of exerting real influence over the problems it tackled. The opportunity came in May, with the publication of 'Primary Health Care in Inner London' (London Health Planning Consortium, 1981). Known as the Acheson Report this was a wide-ranging study of the health care needs of inner London. It had potential implications for all deprived areas of cities in the UK. Among its most interesting comments (buried deep in the body of the report, and—sadly—not mentioned among its recommendations) were the following:

> The identification of the needs of particular communities is essentially a local activity. For each neighbourhood—which may comprise a housing estate, a group of streets, a complex of flats—those responsible for providing health and related social services should meet together on a regular basis. In collaboration with neighbourhood groups and associations, voluntary organisations and representatives of the local community, the professional teams should identify the needs of the population they serve, assess to what extent those needs are being met by existing services, where there are duplications/gaps, or where the introduction of special programmes is required. We believe that effective local planning of this kind will maximise resources available to the community and—in times of severe economic constraints—minimise the effects of a standstill or in some cases cuts in allocated expenditure. It is particularly important, however, both to harness the resources of the community to the full and at the same time provide sufficient professional support so that the demands on local populations do not become burdensome resulting ultimately in complete withdrawal of co-operation.
>
> In some neighbourhoods considerable progress has already been made in this field. Community health workers are providing a stimulus for local discussion and involvement in the planning of health centres, for example, or the development of services for particular groups such as the elderly or mothers and children or the mentally ill. We are aware of projects in Islington, Stockwell, Waterloo, Peckham, Battersea and Deptford for example. We hope to see the example of those communities being developed and extended on a much wider scale.
>
> We recognise, however, that in many neighbourhoods such developments will not come easily. Members of the professions engaged in the delivery of primary health care may not be accustomed to working in collaboration with members of similar yet distinct professions and community identity may be lacking. For this reason, we believe it is necessary for an individual officer to take the initiative in facilitating inter-professional communication and collaboration and community involvement in service provision. As links become established and accepted, we hope that the need for such outside involvement will diminish but initially there will be a need for an officer of fairly senior rank to fulfil this function in each DHA.
>
> (London Health Planning Consortium, 1981, p. 78)

The Acheson Report was considered by the Primary Care subgroup of the Joint Care Planning Team in Liverpool [the JCPT was the officer group which advised the statutory Joint Consultative Committee (JCC) of Liverpool Area

Health Authority (Teaching) and Liverpool City Council]. In November 1981 the JCPT accepted the proposal of the Primary Care subgroup that a pilot Neighbourhood Health Group be established. The adjacent areas of Speke and Garston were chosen. For practical reasons this was subsequently reduced to Speke only.

Establishing the Group

Why had we chosen Speke in which to establish the Neighbourhood Health Group? Speke is a postwar council estate of 18,000 people (1981 census), isolated beyond Liverpool's airport at the south-eastern tip of the city. Unemployment had increased in the decade 1971–1981 from 12 to 30 per cent (compared with a doubling from 10 to 20 per cent in the whole of Liverpool) as many of the purpose-built factories on the Speke Industrial Estate closed down. There are many of the housing types the environmental neglect and the vandalism which characterise the council estates built in many cities in the 1950s and 1960s that are now, prematurely, being rebuilt or demolished. In addition, there was a well-established local concern about health services, focused on the demand for a health centre and minor injuries unit. The estate was remote from the city's major hospitals, the ambulance service was said to be poor and local GPs were reluctant to commit themselves to entering a health centre. The Community Health Council had for some years been co-ordinating and representing these views to the Area Health Authority (AHA) and to the area's MP.

In November 1981 I wrote to all GPs in Speke, to the AHA's community medicine and community nursing managers, to representatives of the City Social Services and Environmental Health Departments, and to the local Council for Voluntary Service, in the following terms:

Neighbourhood Health Group

At its November meeting the Joint Care Planning Team representing Liverpool Area Health Authority (Teaching) and Liverpool City Council agreed to an experimental project whereby a Neighbourhood Health Group should be established and evaluated on a pilot basis.

The principle behind the proposal is very similar to that suggested in the London Health Planning Consortium Report *Primary Health Care in Inner London*. In many areas of deprivation in inner cities it is well established that structural factors relating to the area itself are equally if not more important determinants of health than factors relating to individuals and families. This suggests that a neighbourhood-based approach using the individuals most familiar with the relevant characteristics of the neighbourhood could be profitable in improving the community health. Many such people with this local expertise are already working in parallel with each other, but do not have the opportunity to pool their knowledge.

It is suggested that the Neighbourhood Health Group be established containing the kinds of staff listed below. It may be that in some cases such groups, or elements of them, already exist. Where this is the case then possibly they might be harnessed and/or expanded.

I would be grateful for your comments on this proposal and for suggestions of individuals who could be members of the Neighbourhood Health Group. I would stress that these individuals should be the people actually undertaking the relevant work and not their managers.

I would also be grateful for information about existing groups which may be undertaking the kind of work I have described.

Proposed Representation on Neighbourhood Health Group

General Practitioners
Clinical Medical Officers
Community Nurses
Social Workers
Environmental Health Officers
Voluntary and Community Groups and Workers
Community Health Councils.

A preliminary meeting to establish the NHG was held in Speke in March 1982. Eleven representatives of the groups listed above attended (with the exception of GPs). It was agreed that the general concept of the NHG was worthwhile but that it must 'have teeth' to be effective. It should review specific problems, there should be an open sharing of information between members and agencies, and specific recommendations for change should be made to the health authority and local authority via the JCPT and JCC. The group's terms of reference were agreed as follows:

To consider all aspects, with a bearing on community health, of the policy and delivery of services to the people of Speke and of their social and physical environment; and to make recommendations as appropriate to the Joint Care Planning Team of Liverpool Health Authority and Liverpool City Council.

Major areas of interest for the group's initial discussions were identified as housing (structural problems, vandalism, lack of repairs, and allocation policies), lack of fuel, fuel poverty, diet and nutrition, unemployment, uptake of benefits, social support networks, and health care facilities. Further agencies and individuals were put forward as potential group members. It was agreed to meet every two months, and that the local Social Services office and the Speke Community Council would provide a venue for meetings (subsequently a number of participant agencies provided facilities).

Neighbourhood Health in Action

The Neighbourhood Health Group held its first full meeting in May 1982, following which it met regularly until July 1983. The interest groups represented by the eventual 32 members are shown in Appendix 1. In addition there were *ad hoc* attendances by GPs, housing officers and various other specialist workers when issues of particular relevance to them were discussed. During this

1982–1983 period the attendance was maintained at between 15 and 25. This fact, together with the range and content of the group's activities, gives some indication of its perceived value to participants. These activities are illustrated in the summaries of two of the group's meetings given in Appendix 2. These meetings have been summarised in depth in order to give an idea of how the group worked. These two meetings were mainly concerned with issues relating to housing and the physical environment (both of which the group came to see as crucially important to the local public health) and to health care facilities. However, during its existence the group discussed a much broader range of issues than these; issues that related to the concerns and agencies of every one of its members listed in Appendix 1.

One aspect of the group's functioning that was particularly satisfying was the readiness with which its members accepted, understood and expounded a wide-ranging concept of the public health. They did not need to be told (or to have it 'scientifically proved' to them) that poor nutrition, poverty, lack of education, social isolation or unemployment prevent people living healthy lives. This was most apparent with those working closely with, or suffering the effects of, these conditions. It was equally the norm for all discussions in the group to feature a high level of participation. People far from the health arena, who would not have had much to say on medical matters (like our community policewoman or social security officer), shared an instinctive understanding of the determinants of the public health.

The NHG succeeded in generating participant community action in an area which had seen a wealth of 'community initiatives' come and go. However, given the nature of the group, such success could be achieved only at the expense of creating some controversy in 'establishment' circles. As far as the local authority was concerned, the group's activities and recommendations could be seen as challenging the role of the area's elected representatives. The health authority's lack of enthusiasm was more a function of its orthodox, bureaucratic practice of the 'medical model' of health care. This is a model based essentially on treating diseases in buildings, as compared with a social model of preventing disease—and promoting health—in neighbourhoods.

The Axe

In early 1983, the new District Health Authority in Liverpool was restructuring itself, following the third NHS reorganisation in ten years. Part of this involved a reappraisal of the authority's planning structure. These reorganisations (the fourth occurred in 1984–1985) are fast becoming a way of life in NHS management, as politicians, apparently incapable of experiment and gradual innovation, impose the current managerial 'flavour of the month' in a blanket fashion throughout the service. As well as being very wasteful of NHS resources, disruptive to work and people's lives, they provide a 'legitimate' opportunity for those in power to make unpopular projects or people 'vanish' at the stroke of a pen.

Just such a fate befell the Speke Neighbourhood Health Group. In August 1983, two weeks after a busy meeting at which 15 members discussed the group's proposed primary care survey, antenatal care, the housing repairs service, disconnections and fuel poverty, the health authority's management team decided that the authority 'should no longer have formal involvement with the Neighbourhood Council' (sic). They later informed the Community Health Council that this was because 'the Group had rarely considered Health Service issues, and the Authority already had its own management team which could consider relevant issues'. The Community Health Council quickly stepped in to take over the running of the group, but this withdrawal of its formal links to the health/local authority power structure was a blow from which it never recovered. The Neighbourhood Health Group faded away during the winter of 1983–1984.

The New Public Health

Rather than mourning the passing of the NHG, it is instructive to consider the context in which this occurred. The attitude of the British government to public health issues in the 1980s can be characterised by its handling of the 'Black Report' on inequalities in health (DHSS, 1980). The report's publication was virtually suppressed, and its evidence of widespread social inequalities in health and their implications for social and economic policy was almost totally rejected (Townsend and Davidson, 1982). This political climate has been reflected within the health authorities, whose membership, policies and budgets are strongly influenced by central government. As a result, much of the interest and action in public health issues has occurred outside the NHS. This situation has been reinforced by legislation and government policies (such as on housing, the environment, local authority funding, the abolition of the Greater London and Metropolitan County Councils, privatisation of public sector services, virtual abolition of the school meals service) which have in many areas demonstrably worsened the public health.

In parallel with these events, there has been a major renaissance of public health awareness within local authorities. Beginning with Sheffield in 1981, some 20 councils have established new health committees. In some cases (such as Leeds, Oxford and Lambeth) they have also funded full-time workers or units to develop their public health functions. These include not only the established functions of environmental health and social services, and liaison with the health authority, but also the health implications of the council's housing, education, leisure, transport and planning policies, and its functions as an employer (e.g. providing a healthy working environment, creating socially useful jobs). In the mid 1980s the steady development of these activities has been given extra momentum through the appearance of new 'epidemics': illicit drug use and the acquired immune deficiency syndrome (AIDS), both of which demand a response throughout society. The existence of the 'local authority health network' has assisted substantially in the production of the rapid response required by these 'epidemics'.

A number of local health profiles produced by local authorities have also been important in promoting the new public health (Croxteth Area Working Party, 1983; Thunhurst, 1985; Townsend et al., 1985) and community groups

(Betts, 1985; West of Scotland Politics of Health Group, 1984). These have collated local health and social statistics, undertaken surveys and indicated the actions necessary to address the widespread health inequalities they have identified. Some health authorities have followed suit, though their profiles have tended to be stronger on statistics than on implications for policy (Ashton, 1984; Binysh, Chishty, Middleton and Pollock 1985; Ginnety, Kelly and Black et al., 1985; Sheffield Health Authority, 1986; Townsend et al., 1986).

At the same time, in the non-statutory sector, the community health movement is coming of age. For some years there have been two agencies (the Community Health Initiatives Resource Unit and the London Community Health Resource—now combined as the National Community Health Resource) encouraging and monitoring the accelerating development of community health initiatives, and a number of conferences and publications have resulted (e.g. GLC, 1986; Kenner, 1986; Somerville, 1985). In addition, practical aspects such as the funding and evaluation of projects have received attention (Funding for Health Working Group, 1985; Graessle and Kingsley, 1986; Pollitt, 1984). Despite all this activity it is probably true to say that community health work still remains a relatively unacknowledged approach at the margins of establishment health care.

What little progress there has been within the NHS for the new public health has largely resulted from the actions of a few committed individuals or groups, rather than from any formal policy development process. Examples include experiments with neighbourhood-based ('patch') health care in London (City and Hackney Health Authority, 1985; Dun, 1986) and Norwich (Batch, 1986) and an excellent report from the Scottish Health Education Co-ordinating Committee (1984). However, two recent events are helping to strengthen the statutory response. The first was the production by the European Region of the World Health Organization (WHO) of 'Targets for Health for All' (WHO, 1985) in support of its strategy of 'health for all by the year 2000'. The British government endorsed the 38 targets of the WHO in 1984 and, though any practical effects of this action have been slow in emerging (Draper and Scott-Samuel, 1986), it seems that something is beginning to happen. The WHO strategy takes the major elements of the new public health (equity, community participation, intersectoral collaboration, primary health care and health promotion) as its basis, and the NHS annual report for 1985–1986 tells us that 'the Government strongly supports this Strategy' (DHSS, 1986).

The other important spur to action has been the government's Community Nursing Review (Cumberlege Report) which proposes the organisation of all community nurses into neighbourhood teams (DHSS, 1986). While this would not of itself have truly radical effects, the principle of NHS Neighbourhood Health Teams which it establishes creates an important potential for developing the 'patch' approach in health care. Elsewhere (Scott-Samuel, 1986), I have proposed using this principle to create Neighbourhood Prevention Teams (based on health visitors, community health doctors and environmental health officers) which would work in a way broadly comparable to that of the Speke Neighbourhood Health Group in promoting the local public health. These teams could be created overnight with little or no cost or disruption.

Postscript

And what of Speke? Even ill winds blow some good and, three years after the demise of the Neighbourhood Health Group, things have begun to change. An assertive local Women's Health Action Group has unexpectedly succeeded where others have failed in prevailing on the District Health Authority (DHA) and Family Practitioner Committee (FPC) to agree to build a health centre. A spin-off of the independence granted to FPCs by the government in 1985 has been the appointment of a development worker to stimulate and evaluate DHA/FPC collaboration in primary health care in Speke. It seems that a number of helpful health care developments will emerge from this initiative. While it may be a long time before the new public health becomes the order of the day and percolates through the baroque structures of NHS management to the many estates and people who have not shared the 'good fortune' of Speke, something at least, at last, is happening.

References

Ashton, J. (1984) *Health in Mersey—a Review.* Department of Community Health, University of Liverpool, Liverpool.

Batch, C. (1986) 'Community Care Groups', *Radical Health Promotion*, No. 3 (Winter), 21–22.

Betts, G. (1985) *Health in Glyndon.* Greenwich Health Rights Project, London.

Binysh, K., Chishty, V., Middleton, J., and Pollock, G. (1985) *The Health of Coventry.* Coventry Health Authority, Coventry.

City and Hackney Health Authority (1985) *Patch Based Care—Organising Primary Care in the Community Health Services in City and Hackney Health District.* City and Hackney Health Authority, London.

Croxteth Area Working Party (1983) *Report.* City Solicitor's Department, Liverpool City Council, Liverpool.

Department of Health and Social Security (1980) *Inequalities in Health. Report of a Research Working Group.* DHSS, London.

Department of Health and Social Security (1986) *The Health Service in England. Annual Report 1985–6.* DHSS, London.

Department of Health and Social Security (1986) *Neighbourhood Nursing—a Focus for Care. Report of the Community Nursing Review.* HMSO, London. (Cumberlege Report.)

Draper, P., and Scott-Samuel, A. (1986) 'Whatever happened to Public Health?' *Health Service Journal*, 6 March, 322–323.

Dun, R. (1986) *PATCH—Primary Action Towards Community Health.* West Lambeth Health Authority, London.

Funding for Health Working Group (1985) *Funding for Health Resource Pack.* London Community Health Resource and Community Health Initiatives Resource Unit, London.

Ginnety, P., Kelly, K., and Black, M. (1985) *Moyard : a Health Profile*, Parts 1 and 2. Eastern Health and Social Services Board, Belfast.

Greater London Council (1986) *Innovation in Everyday Health Care—the Conference Papers.* King's Fund Centre, London.

Graessle, L., and Kingsley, S. (1986) *Measuring Change, Making Changes—an Approach to Evaluation.* London Community Health Resource, London.

Kenner, C. (1986) *Whose Needs Count? Community Action for Health*. Bedford Square Press, London.

London Health Planning Consortium (1981) *Primary Health Care in Inner London*. LHPC, London. (Acheson Report.)

Pollitt, C. (1984) *An Evaluation of the Community Health Projects at Walker, North Kenton and Riverside*. Riverside Child Health Project, Newcastle.

Scottish Health Education Co-ordinating Committee (1984) *Health Education in Areas of Multiple Deprivation*. Scottish Home and Health Department, Edinburgh.

Scott-Samuel, A. (1986) 'A new public health practice', *Radical Community Medicine*, No. 27 (Autumn), 4–6

Sheffield Health Authority (1986) *Health Care and Disease—a Profile of Sheffield*. Sheffield Health Authority, Sheffield.

Somerville, G. (1985) *Community Development in Health: Addressing the Confusions*. King's Fund Centre, London.

Thunhurst, C. (1985) *Poverty and Health in the City of Sheffield*. Environmental Health Department, Sheffield City Council, Sheffield.

Townsend, P., and Davidson, N. (eds) (1982) *Inequalities in Health. The Black Report*. Penguin Books, Harmondsworth.

Townsend, P., Simpson, D., and Tibbs, N. (1985) 'Inequalities in Health in the City of Bristol: A Preliminary Review of Statistical Evidence', *International Journal of Health Services*, **15**, 637–663.

Townsend, P., Phillimore, P., and Beattie, A. (1986) *Inequalities in Health in the Northern Region*. Northern Regional Health Authority and University of Bristol, Bristol.

Unit for the Study of Health Policy (1979) *Rethinking Community Medicine*. USHP, London.

Watt, A. (1986) 'Community Health Initiatives and Their Relationship to General Practice', *Journal of the Royal College of General Practitioners*, **36**, 72–73.

West of Scotland Politics of Health Group (1984) *Glasgow: Health of a City*. WSPOHG, Glasgow.

World Health Organization (1978) 'Declaration of Alma-Ata', *Lancet*, **2**, 1040–1041.

World Health Organization (1985) *Targets for Health for All*. WHO Regional Office for Europe, Copenhagen.

Appendix 1. Speke Neighbourhood Health Group— Membership

Health authority

1. Community Health Services	Senior clinical medical officer School medical officer Nursing officer—health visiting Nursing officer—district nursing School nurse
2. Community medicine	Community physician Trainee community physician (senior registrar)

Local authority

1. Social services	District officer
	Two social workers
	Senior occupational therapist
	Health liaison officer (from Social Services Department)
2. Environmental health	Senior public health inspector
3. Housing	District housing manager
4. Education	Head teacher (infants' school)
	Education welfare officer
	Community education officer
	Education guidance officer
Community health council	Secretary
	Two local members (including one vicar)
Voluntary/community groups	Citizens' Advice Bureau
	Age Concern
	Crescent 73 Mental Health Association
	Speke Community Council
	Speke Enterprise Centre
	Speke Together Action Resource
DHSS	Liaison officer
Probation	Two probation officers
Police	Community police constable
Media	*Speke Press*

Appendix 2. Speke Neighbourhood Health Group—Summaries of Meetings held in July 1982 and March 1983

July 1982

Information circulated

Letter from Chief Ambulance Officer giving results of survey of response times to emergency calls from Speke.

Funding proposals to Inner City Partnership (ICP) for (i) study of primary care needs of deprived areas; (ii) Family Centre in Speke.

Discussion topics/actions

Issues arising from minibus tour of Speke (undertaken in June):

1. Under-use of public baths due to financial barriers. *Action*—request to City Council to list existing subsidies on leisure facilities and to introduce comprehensive policy of subsidies for all state benefit recipients and their dependants.
2. Rubbish accumulation behind flats and houses; in blocked chutes in flats; in Speke Market adjacent to Day Nursery. *Action*—request to City Council to declare overall cleansing policy for Speke, and to place skips in areas where existing facilities inadequate.
3. Tenants in 'walk-up' flats are themselves responsible for gardens around flats. Elderly tenants unable to cut grass, which becomes rubbish trap. *Action*—request to City Council to accept responsibilty for gardens.

Community Policewoman member of NHG to follow up possibility of producing local crime statistics.

Ambulance callout survey discussed. *Action*—further information requested: to include numbers of 'inappropriate' calls e.g. for primary care, or because no personal transport to hospital available.

ICP research proposal. *Action*—recommendation that if funded this be undertaken in Speke. Agreed also to approach a local pharmaceutical company to fund such a study; and to set up a working group to design it.

ICP Family Centre proposal (support centre for families with identified or potential parenting problems). *Action*—recommendation that the Health Authority support the proposal.

Senior clinic doctor reported proposal to Health Authority for local paediatric clinic facilities to be provided.

Housing Manager described current year's programme for conversion of unsuitable flats into houses/bungalows.

March 1983

Information circulated

Proposed primary care survey—initial list of health needs and problem areas identified by NHG members as basis for survey.

Report from School Medical Service re minor ailment clinics.

Letters from City Solicitor (Secretary to City Council) re (i) NHG recommendations on Schools' Hair Cleansing Service; (ii) NHG recommendations on Housing Repairs Service, Maintenance of Open Spaces, Tenant Participation in Housing Policy, Default Power of Chief Environmental Health Officer; (iii) NHG recommendations on Use of Leisure Facilites by the Unemployed.

Letter from Family Practitioner Committee re adequacy of GP premises.

Discussion topics/actions

Primary care survey. An initial 'trawl' of NHG members had produced a range of local public health issues on which to base a survey. A funding source had not yet been identified and it was agreed to approach Speke Together, the Community Health Council and the Health Authority.

Minor Ailments Clinic. The group felt that much inappropriate care occurred locally as a result of the closure of this service (e.g. some minor treatments were being carried out by school ancillary workers; anti-tetanus injections often not being given when required). *Action*—request to Health Authority to consider reopening School Minor Ailments Clinic in Speke.

Hair Cleansing Service for schoolchildren. Group pleased to note that this was being reinstated in response to its recommendation.

GP premises. The group noted that all local GP premises (which it had previously discussed) did meet DHSS guidelines on numbers of seats in waiting rooms. However they felt that these guidelines were inadequate in that they made no reference to heating of waiting rooms or to the seating needs of the children of single parents and large families.

Housing and health. The group agreed to the City Solicitor's suggestion that it monitor the recently reviewed Housing Repairs Service. It noted that he had requested the Director of Recreation and Open Spaces and the Chief Environmental Health Officer to liaise concerning the maintenance of grassed areas around the flats. It declined his suggestion that the NHG should advise on tenant participation in housing policy—this was a function of the Housing Department and local tenants' organisations. The City Solicitor had expressed satisfaction with the scheme whereby the Chief Environmental Health Officer served 'informal notices' on the Housing Department where there were urgent structural problems in council housing. The group requested evidence regarding the effectiveness of this process.

Subsidised leisure facilities. The group was pleased to hear that the City Council was making its leisure facilities more freely available to unemployed people, but repeated its recommendations regarding other benefit recipients and the dependants of all of these groups.

Chapter Six
Liverpool: Creating a Healthy City*

JOHN ASHTON
Senior Lecturer in Community Health
University of Liverpool
UK

Introduction

The Healthy Cities Project is a European World Health Organization initiative that is intended to lend support to health promotion in cities. Throughout Europe there is a renaissance of public health activity in cities, and it is appropriate that the WHO are supporting and facilitating processes that are already under way.

The project, which is being co-ordinated from Liverpool University, is bringing together a group of European cities to collaborate in the implementation of intersectoral city health plans. By concentrating on concrete examples of health promotion it is expected that the Healthy Cities Project will mark the point at which WHO philosophies and frameworks are taken off the shelves and into the streets of European cities.

The Healthy Cities Project contains three major elements:

1. The formulation of concepts to provide a solid rationale for action to create health in cities.
2. The implementation and monitoring of good practice.
3. The dissemination of ideas and experiences between collaborating cities.

The success of the project within Merseyside and throughout Europe will depend upon two factors. First, it will be necessary to draw upon the new concepts and approaches to health promotion that have become known as 'the new public health'. Second, it will be necessary to build upon the experience that some of the larger cities have already had in developing new health promotion initiatives. The concepts and practices stretch across conventional boundaries and sectors. The ultimate plan is that a comprehensive approach

---

*This chapter contains short extracts from the book *The New Public Health*, by J. Ashton and H. Seymour, Open University Press, 1988, reproduced with permission.

to health promotion should incorporate all aspects of city life, including architecture, transport and recreation as well as employment, housing, education and medical care.

This chapter examines the background to and prospects for Healthy Cities work in the Mersey region. The first section looks at some principles of the new public health, and the second describes initiatives already undertaken in the region.

The Evolution of the New Public Health

It is helpful when trying to understand the present trends to place them in context. The public health movement grew up in industrial towns and cities during the nineteenth century. The situation then was more clear-cut than it is today. There seemed to be little point in discussing definitions of health when as many as a third of new-born infants failed to survive to their first birthday. Mortality rates from the infectious disease epidemics such as cholera, typhoid, smallpox and infantile diarrhoea proved to be sufficient to focus attention on the necessity for very specific interventions and public health legislation. Early medical officers of health, such as Duncan in Liverpool and Snow in London, were able to draw on the sense of urgency that was present in relation to infectious disease to obtain support for their work. This sense of imperative has, until recently, been lacking with respect to the non-infectious diseases and lifestyle problems such as heart disease, stroke, cancers, accidents and suicide, which characterise present-day populations.

The continuing power of the fear of infection can be seen clearly in the present level of activity that has arisen in response to AIDS, which seems to have breathed new life into some old and apparently moribund public health institutions.

One of the tensions between the old and the new approaches to public health is between 'paternalism' and 'participation'. The potential conflict inherent in every public health issue between individual and collective liberty is particularly acute with infectious disease, where one person's behaviour may lead to another's illness. The situation is less clear-cut with individual behaviour in relation to the non-infectious diseases, where the effects are less direct. The effect of the apparently simple cause and effect relationship associated with infection has been that in the past the public appeared to be willing to accept restrictions on personal liberty, for example through compulsory notification of infectious disease and quarantine provisions, whereas today support for the same course of action in response to AIDS would by no means be universal. It may be that the mass of the population is less willing today than it was in the 1840s and 1850s to tolerate paternalistic as opposed to collaborative and participative responses. In time, the public health movement of the last century was eclipsed by a more individualistic medical approach. As the most pressing environmental problems were brought under control, action to improve the health of the population moved on. The focus first moved to personal, preventive medical services, such as immunisation and the monitoring of growth and development of schoolchildren, and later to clinical therapeutics spurred on by the discovery of antibiotics (Kickbusch, 1986; Acheson, 1988). What is curious is that until comparatively recently many people, both professional and lay, seem to have subscribed to the view that the dramatic improvements in health that have been achieved in developed countries have occurred as a result of advances in scientific and laboratory medicine. Since about 1970 this view has increasingly been challenged, not least by Thomas McKeown as a result of his analysis of changes in death rates and population growth in England and Wales since 1840 (McKeown, 1976). According to McKeown, during most of the history of the human race a large proportion of all children probably died or were killed in the first few years of life. It seems that the high death rates of the past were mainly caused by infectious disease in populations that were vulnerable because of the effects of poverty, which led to poor nutrition and insanitary environments.

McKeown has suggested that between 80 and 90 per cent of the total reduction in the death rate during the past 150 years has been brought about by a reduction in those deaths caused by infection. The most important of these have been tuberculosis, chest infections and the water- and food-borne diarrhoeal diseases.

McKeown's analysis is striking for its conclusion that with the exception of vaccination against smallpox it is unlikely that immunisation and treatment had much effect on death rates before the present century. In particular, most of the reduction in deaths from tuberculosis, bronchitis, pneumonia, influenza, whooping cough and water- and food-borne disease had already occurred before effective immunisation and treatments were available. In effect, the total contribution of medical and surgical action on reductions in death rates has been small compared with the effect of environmental, political, economic and social measures. It seems clear that in order of importance the major contributions to improvements in health have stemmed from limitation of family size, increases in the quality and quantity of food supplies, and a healthier physical environment. Specific preventive medicine and treatment appears lower on the list.

When the present pattern of illness is analysed it is immediately noticeable that much of it is preventable and that it affects a comparatively small proportion of the population (excluding the elderly population).

Preventive medicine and health promotion have begun to combine the approach that identifies the causes of premature death in individuals with the approach that starts from social factors. The former has highlighted accidents and the consequences of tobacco use, alcohol misuse, a diet that is high in fat and low in fibre, and a failure to take regular exercise. The latter has identified the importance of planned parenthood and a good start in life, good living and working conditions, an environment that enhances health and well-being, the prospects for satisfying work, non-exploitative and fulfilling personal relationships, and the realisation of abilities. This approach explains how the absence of these factors can play a part in generating a whole range of health problems, including emotional disorders, alcohol and drug abuse, rejected and abused children, violence, antisocial behaviour, and suicide.

The new public health is based upon social as well as biological aspects of health. Many contemporary health problems are seen as inherently social rather than individual, with underlying concrete issues of local and national public policy (Milio, 1986).

The European programme of Health for All (WHO, 1985) is intended to achieve a shift away from a narrow medical view of health towards a fuller appreciation of the social determinants of health.

At the 1986 Ottawa conference on health promotion certain principles were developed as the 'Ottawa Charter for Health Promotion' (WHO, 1986). This charter stresses in particular the necessity to:

1. Build public policies that support health — Health promotion goes beyond conventional health care and makes health an agenda item for policy makers in all areas of governmental and organisational action. Health promotion requires that the obstacles to the adoption of health promoting policies be identified in non-medical sectors together with ways of removing them. The aim must be to make the healthier choices the easier choices.
2. Create supportive environments — Health promotion recognises that both at the global level and at the local level human health is bound up with the way in which we treat nature and the environment. Societies that exploit their environments without attention to ecology, reap the effects of that exploitation in ill-health and social problems. Health cannot be separated from other goals and changing patterns of life. Work and leisure have a definite impact on health. Health promotion, therefore, must create living and working conditions that are safe, stimulating, satisfying and enjoyable.
3. Strengthen community action — Health promotion works through effective community action. At the heart of this process is the need for communities to have power and control of their own initiatives and activities. This means that professionals must learn new ways of working with individuals and communities — working for and with them rather than on them.
4. Develop personal skills — Health promotion supports personal and social development by providing information and education for health, and by helping people to develop the skills that they need to make healthy choices. By doing so it enables people to exercise more control over their health and their environments. It is essential to make it possible for people to learn throughout life, to prepare themselves for all of its stages and to cope with chronic illness and injuries. This has to be assisted in school, home, work and in community settings.
5. Reorientate health services — The responsibility for health promotion in health services is shared between community groups, health professionals, medical carers, bureaucracies and governments. They must work together towards a health care system that contributes to the pursuit of health. The role of the medical sector must develop beyond its responsibility to provide treatment services to include health promotion. To do this it will need to recognise that most of the causes of ill-health lie outside the direct influence of the medical sector and be willing to work with those in a position to influence these factors.

Public Health in the Mersey Region — A Case Study

The Mersey Regional Health Authority covers two counties in the north-west of England and is responsible for hospital medical and community care services, excepting general practice, for 2.4 million people. Beginning from a low base of health promotion activity in 1983 a regional strategy for health promotion has been developed based on the concepts and principles of Health for All.

The first step was to establish a multi-disciplinary Regional Health Promotion Team within the health authority (Ashton, 1982). The most important initial function of this team was to obtain access to the range of resources that exist within health authorities and to open up channels of communication for influencing policy making. Beginning with very modest resources a Regional Health Promotion Unit has been established. By achieving a high public visibility and demonstrating results it has grown into an important and influential section of the health authority, with a management steering group constituted as a sub-committee of the health authority itself.

Agenda setting

A reference point for some of the recent Mersey health promotion initiatives is the community diagnosis produced in 1983–1984: *Health in Mersey — A Review* (Ashton, 1984). This 91-page document assesses the state of health of people in the Mersey region, making comparisons between the ten districts. It was written particularly for the informed lay reader, and was targeted at decision-makers and opinion-formers within the region. In all, more than 6000 copies have been distributed to date, a large proportion of them on my request. This document has played a part in two processes — it has informed the strategies developed by the regional and district health authorities, and has also informed the public. The review was launched at the first Mersey regional health promotion conference, a one-day event attended by 550 key opinion-formers and decision-makers. This led to the inclusion of a table of priorities for action in the regional strategic plan.

The priorities and strategies have been subject to monitoring and review and, with hindsight, the original list can be seen to have some limitations. They have sometimes been criticised for being too wide-ranging, encompassing as they do clinical preventive activity, environmental health protection and very far-reaching policy issues relating to such things as youth alienation and unemployment. However, the initiative began from a fairly conventional medical approach to public health. As the work develops, the importance of social and anthropological factors has become ever more apparent, particularly as a result of specific project work. As entry points to health promotion strategies the 12 priorities have been effective. They have been particularly useful in ensuring that health promotion is taken seriously. The danger lies in their generally reductionist and medical nature, which might distract attention from the need for horizontal, integrative, participative and intersectoral strategies.

Consciousness raising

A well-informed public is the counterpart to a well-briefed executive and bureaucracy. To achieve this it is necessary to have in parallel with the agenda setting a process of consciousness raising on a large scale. Such consciousness raising needs to be much more than classroom education, posters and leaflets, or even television advertising. To be effective it needs to employ many varied methods and is likely to be most powerful when it addresses the issues that most affect the public. One element of such an approach is the health fair as an opportunity for active learning (Hussey, *et al.*, 1987).

The International Garden Festival, held in Liverpool from April to October 1984, offered a unique opportunity to provide information for a mass audience as part of Mersey Regional Health Authority's health promotion strategy. Health was made a major theme throughout the festival. Educational material was featured in a number of areas within the site, including the area containing allotments and domestic gardens. The term 'health fair' was used to denote the range of activities rather than describe a single static base. The objective was to provide active learning. Activities included static displays, which provided information on a range of health matters, dynamic displays, which included aerobic dancing, yoga, meditation and sports; and public participation which involved physical fitness testing and interactive computerised lifestyle assessment.

It is estimated that a quarter of a million of the 3.3 million people who attended the International Garden Festival attended the static part of the fair, and most of them made use of the computerised lifestyle assessment — 11,000 actually took a fitness test. Software was developed for computer analysis of lifestyle and fitness, and this has subsequently been in steady demand both at home and abroad.

Part of the hidden health promotion agenda was to provide positive work experience for the 56 long-term unemployed people who were recruited to staff the health fair as part of a Manpower Services Commission Community Programme. The staff had the opportunity to be part of a friendly but task-orientated work-group with a great deal of public contact and potential job satisfaction. In addition, they gained a great deal of health knowledge for themselves and their families. A high proportion of the staff obtained work during the period of the scheme, and some returned to study having found renewed self-confidence and motivation. Arrangements were made for staff to receive details of National Health Service vacancies that occurred whilst they were on the scheme.

The importance of an emphasis on personal development in such schemes as part of a health promotion strategy is self-evident, and efforts are now being made to extend the possiblities through scheme exchanges with other countries. Job creation is in itself a health promotion priority in an area where some local government wards have as many as 80 per cent of the adult males unemployed.

The opportunist use of publicity and of the mass media, and many other examples of small-scale innovations and projects that involve public participation, provide for consciousness raising on a continuing basis.

Examples of good practice

The attempt to develop and disseminate models of good practice is essential to the new public health. This approach has been used in Mersey to identify and make explicit the key principles of health promotion.

1. The Health and Recreation Team (HART)   A Sports-Council-funded project, based initially in one health centre, was inspired by the Peckham Pioneer Health Centre, which was founded in prewar London (Ashton, 1977). That centre was a social experiment that sought to influence the environmental and behavioural determinants of health. The Peckham Pioneer Health Centre failed to achieve the necessary support for its continuation when the National Health Service was established in 1948, partly because it did not accord with contemporary wisdom about the role of medical care, which was seen as becoming increasingly therapeutic.

The sort of comprehensive social, education and health centre run on co-operative lines, as pioneered in Peckham, is unlikely to be established today in a new building. However, it is possible to consider related community resources, such as community centres, sports centres and various education and training centres as potentially part of a 'networked health centre' — a functional rather than a physical concept. It should be possible to enter any of these public institutions and readily gain access to the services in the others. The HART project employs a community development worker to develop these networks, particularly as they relate to sport and exercise. In Liverpool, extensive and active links have now been developed between a number of health and community centres and local government and non-governmental organisations, as a result of the project (Ireland, 1985). HART has given a considerable boost to the local 'Look After Yourself!' programme, has produced a comprehensive local survey of exercise participation, and has developed a number of other initiatives including group outings of women from one health centre for swimming classes at the local baths; rambling in the Welsh mountains for inner city health centre children; and support for collaborative fun-runs with community groups. It thus provides support for community involvement and organisation.

2. Merseyside Drugs Information and Training Centre   The centre offers a free information service for professional staff and the general public. This includes a wide range of literature on the nature and effects of drug misuse. It also houses a library of up-to-date research reports. In addition training is available, not only for professional workers, but also for voluntary and parent support groups. It has been so successful that similar centres are now being established on a district basis and it has been able to move on to further innovative work. Recent initiatives include the first syringe-exchange scheme for drug users. This has revealed a previously unrecognised population of intravenous drug users. Free condoms are provided for drug users, as well as for a regular clientele of local prostitutes.

3. Urban horticulture   In the inner city areas of Mersey region, issues of employment, environment, housing, poverty and health converge. The population of the city of Liverpool has decreased by 20 per cent over the past 15 years. The adult male unemployment rate is currently about 28 per cent. Deserted factories, abandoned land and slum housing are characteristic of some of the inner city wards. The Regional Health Promotion Unit has been collaborating with The Eldonians (a community-based housing co-operative), housing associations, the government task force and various other agencies to develop a community business to use derelict land for urban horticulture. This project is at an advanced stage of planning, and has given rise to other ideas about the potential for creating new jobs in relation to 'healthy products'.

The work with the Eldonians, perhaps more than any other of the Regional Health Promotion Unit's initiatives, has underlined the importance of starting from people's own priorities. For the Eldonians their immediate priorities are housing and jobs. Their attitude to professionals is best summarised by their belief that professionals should be 'on tap not on top'.

Future work is to include a community centred health survey, which will enable the community association to produce its own corporate plan for local health.

4. A health promotion information service   During 1985–1986, Mersey Regional Health Promotion Unit piloted a health promotion information service, which the region and districts agreed to fund for a further three years. This information service supports individuals within the region who are working to set up or develop health promotion initiatives. Enquirers are helped with up-to-date information and contacts in their areas of interest. Negotiations have begun with other regions and interested organisations to see if existing or planned health promotion information services could form a collaborative network whereby each service would be able to provide a broader and more cost-effective service to its own clients.

5. The Mind, Body, City Museum   A development of the health fair — the Mind, Body, City Museum is a joint project under discussion between the Mersey Regional Health Authority and Merseyside Development Corporation. It is intended to draw in the leisure industry and commercial organisations. (Seymour, Ashton and Edwards, 1986). The museum would be something between a science centre and a theme park. It would aim to give people a powerful and enjoyable insight into the workings of their own bodies and minds. It would use the best ideas and technology of the modern museum and the theme park industry, and it would create jobs in an area of high unemployment.

Conclusion

Innovation is never easy. In developing participative, intersectoral health promotion that has a distinct social entrepreneurial style, there have been many times when a health authority has not seemed to be the most appropriate base.

The history of British health authorities lies with hospital management by appointed members, rather than with politically-responsive, broadly-based local initiatives from the Town Hall. In Commonwealth countries that have retained the British model of a local authority public health department (e.g. Canada), the potential for developing an effective new public health seems exceptionally rich. Local government in Toronto, for instance, has the aim of making Toronto the healthiest city in North America by the year 2000 (Ashton, Grey and Barnard, 1986). However, despite the difficulties, there is within the Mersey region a real commitment to developing health promotion.

References

Acheson, E. D. (1988) 'On the State of the Nation's Health, Fourth Duncan Memorial Lecture, Liverpool' *Public Health*, **102**, 431–437.

Ashton, J. (1977) 'The Peckham Pioneer Health Centre: a Reappraisal', *Community Health*, **8**, 132–137.

Ashton, J. (1982) 'Towards Prevention — an Outline Plan for the Development of Health Promotion Teams', *Community Medicine*, **4**, 231–237.

Ashton, J. (1984) *Health in Mersey — a Review*. University of Liverpool, Deparment of Community Health, Liverpool.

Ashton, J. (1985a) 'Health in Mersey — an Exercise in Community Diagnosis'. *Health Education Journal*, **44**, 178–180.

Ashton, J. (1985b) 'Pollution of the Water Supply in Mersey and Clwyd — a Cause for Concern?' *Community Medicine*, **7**, 229–303.

Ashton, J., Grey P. and Barnard, K. (1986) 'Health Cities — WHO's New Public Health Initiative', *Health Promotion* **1**, 319–324.

Ashton, J., Seymour, H., Ingledew, D., Ireland, R., Hopley, E., Parry, A., Ryan, M., and Holbourn, A. (1986) 'Promoting the New Public Health in Mersey', *Health Education Journal*, **45**, 174–179.

Chadwick, E., (1842) *Report on the Sanitary Conditions of the Labouring Population of Great Britain*. Republished by Edinburgh University Press, Edinburgh (1965) (ed. M. W. Flinn).

Chave, S. P. W. (1955) 'The Broad Street Pump and After', *The Medical Officer*, **99**, 347–349.

Chave, S. P. W. (1984) 'Duncan of Liverpool — and Some Lessons for Today', *Community Medicine*, **6**, 61–71.

Godber, G. E. (1986) 'Medical Officers of Health and Health Services', *Community Medicine*, **8**, 1–14.

Hellberg, H. (1987) 'Health for All and Primary Health Care in Europe', *Public Health* **101**, 151–157.

Hussey, R. M., Edwards, M. B., Reid, J. A., Sykes, K., Seymour, H., Hopley, E., Ashton, J. R. (1987) 'Evaluation of the International Garden Festival Health Fair, Liverpool 1984'. *Public Health* **101**, 111–117.

Ingledew, D. (1986) *A Review of the Health Promotion Activities of the District Health Authorities of Mersey Region*. Mersey Regional Health Authority, Liverpool.

Ireland, R. (1985) *Health and Recreation Team (HART)*, Mersey Regional Health Authority Phase 1 Monitoring Report — Establishing the Project. Sports Council Research Unit, Liverpool.

Kickbusch, I. (1986) 'Health Promotion: a Global perspective', *Canadian Journal of Public Health*, **77**, 321–326.

Lalonde, M. (1974) *A New Perspective on the Health of Canadians*. Minister of Supply and Services.

McKeown, T. (1976) *The Role of Medicine, Dream, Mirage or Nemesis?* Nuffield Provincial Hospital Trust.

Milio, N. (1986) *Promoting Health through Public Policy*. Canadian Public Health Association, Ottawa.

Seedhouse, D. (1986) *Health: The Foundations for Achievement*. John Wiley, Chichester.

Seymour, H., Ashton, J. and Edwards, P. (1986) 'Health Museums or Theme Parks: a New Approach to Intersectoral Collaboration', *Health Promotion* **1**, 311–317.

Snow, J. (1855) *On the Mode of Communication of Cholera* (2nd edn). Churchill, London.

World Health Organization, (1981) *Global Strategy for Health for All by the Year 2000*. WHO, Geneva.

World Health Organization (1984) *Health Promotion. A discussion document on the concept and principles*, ICP/HSR 602 (mol). WHO, Copenhagen.

World Health Organization (1985) *Targets for Health for All*. WHO Regional Office for Europe.

World Health Organization (1986) *Ottawa. Charter for Health Promotion*. WHO, Copenhagen.

Changing Ideas in Health Care
Edited by D. Seedhouse and A. Cribb
© 1989 John Wiley & Sons Ltd

Chapter Seven
'Heartbeat Wales': New Horizons for Health Promotion in the Community — the Philosophy and Practice of Heartbeat Wales

JOHN CATFORD AND RICHARD PARISH
Heartbeat Wales
Cardiff
UK

Introduction

This chapter illustrates the concept of health promotion in practice in the UK by examining the project 'Heartbeat Wales'. The first section outlines the enterprise and the implications of this as a demonstration project for the UK. The intervention frameworks are then presented, followed by a description of the Choice–Change–Champion process for health promotion, developed as a tool to guide planning and priority setting in Wales. The following sections describe the practical programmes of action that have been mounted and their effect in achieving change through public affairs and mass communication, health authorities, primary health care, community groups and voluntary organisations, schools and young people, local authorities, the workplace, and industry and commerce.

Background to Heartbeat Wales

The Welsh Heart Programme is a major national demonstration project to promote good health amongst the three-million population in Wales. It is particularly concerned with reducing the risks of cardiovascular disease throughout the whole of the Principality. Its major priorities include the encouragement of non-smoking, creating habits of good nutrition, facilitating and promoting regular exercise, the management of stress, and the provision of health screening and first aid for heart attacks. The long-term aim of the programme is to develop and evaluate, as a pilot venture, a regional strategy that will contribute to a sustained reduction in the incidence of coronary heart disease, morbidity and mortality in the general population of Wales, and in particular those under the age of 65.

The programme was publicly launched on St David's Day, 1 March 1985, in response to the high incidence of coronory heart disease in the Principality, for an initial five-year period as 'Curiad Calon Cymru/Heartbeat Wales', and has since attracted considerable lay, professional, political and media interest (Parish, Catford and Nutbeam, 1987). Initially, core funding was provided by the Health Education Council and the Welsh Office, and the project was administered through the University of Wales College of Medicine. The Welsh Health Promotion Authority took over the funding responsibilities on 1 April 1987. Considerable additional support is also provided by statutory, commercial and voluntary agencies as well as the general public in Wales.

Generating initial local support

The importance of participation by the many communities in Wales was recognised at the outset. Considerable energy, therefore, was directed to meeting key individuals and agencies throughout Wales during the early months, in order to plan a programme that would meet the interests of Welsh people and generate support. This culminated in the publication of a detailed consultative document, *Take Heart* (WHPD, 1985) which outlined the proposed strategy and described the conceptual framework. The document generated an overwhelming response from health authorities, community health councils, family practitioner committees, individual health professionals, voluntary agencies, county councils, national and local politicians, and district and borough councils. Almost without exception the comments supported the proposed strategy.

Evaluating the project

The project is to be evaluated by a number of methods (Nutbeam and Catford, 1987). To plan and evaluate the programme it is necessary to have recent and relevant population-based information on individuals, their lifestyles and risk factors. Such information is not available in any comprehensive form from regularly collected government statistics. To meet this information gap the Welsh Heart Health Surveys were planned and carried out during 1985 and 1986. The report *Pulse of Wales* (WHPD, 1986a) contains a summary of the key information for Wales derived from an initial analysis of a large questionnaire survey (The 'Community Survey') of 22,000 Welsh people aged 12–64 who were randomly selected from the electoral register. Subsequent reports include information collected from medical examinations (the 'Clinical Survey'), and a special survey of young people (the 'Youth Survey'). The large database for Wales allows analysis of the health status of the population area by area. Individual reports for each county and health authority have been produced together with a special social survey supplement.

As well as assessing the outcome of the intervention, great emphasis is also placed on process evaluation; on how and why the changes were achieved. The evaluation strategy for the programme (Nutbeam and Catford, 1987) sets out a number of approaches, one of which includes measuring organisational change, particularly in hospitals, schools and the workplace. Other evaluation projects include a study of opinion leaders, a series of market research surveys and a network of consumer panels across Wales.

Intervention Frameworks

The programme was set up as a community-based project drawing substantially on intrinsic resources from within the varied communities and organisations in Wales. As a consequence the intervention comprises a wide range of locally organised projects together with centrally led initiatives. A broad range of approaches to health education and health promotion are being used across all sectors of Welsh life.

Suggested goals for the programme were presented in *Take Heart*. They include not only targeted reductions in mortality, morbidity and population risk factors for coronary heart disease, but also changes in related health behaviours, attitudes and knowledge. The promotion of a healthy lifestyle is at the core of the project, and an important part of the strategy is to achieve environmental, organisational, structural and policy changes within Wales that will support healthy choices. Targets include restricting smoking in public places, better food labelling, price incentives, increasing availability of 'healthy' foods in shops, workplace canteens and restaurants, and changing work practices amongst health and education professionals.

In developing an intervention strategy the experiences of other community-based cardiovascular risk reduction programmes have been drawn on, particularly the North Karelia Project in Finland and the Stanford, Minnesota and Pawtucket heart disease prevention programmes in the USA (Blackburn et al., 1984; Farquhar et al., 1984; Lasater et al., 1984; Puska et al., 1985). The main intervention approaches to be used in the Welsh initiative are outlined below.

Social learning

The application of social learning theory (Bandura, 1977) places health education activity in a social setting and stresses the importance of external factors in behaviour change. The promotion of healthy role models or exemplars at the local level and in the media has been an early priority of the programme. For example, several 'healthy living' television programmes have been co-produced by Heartbeat Wales and broadcast at peak viewing times to large numbers of Welsh people. The development of personal *skill* as well as the *will* to change receives high priority in health education activities. Feelings of self-empowerment and self-efficacy are crucial for success in individual behavioural change. Promoting *self-esteem* and *self-confidence* by positive messages, through personal or mass media health education, are therefore fundamental concerns.

Community development

Health promotion through community development enables and facilitates existing community networks and resources to achieve health goals. This has been an important component of the North Karelia, Minnesota and Pawtucket projects (Bracht et al., 1987; Lasater et al., 1984; Tuomilehto et al., 1983). This approach has been adapted to the Welsh situation, and national networks such as the Women's Institute and the Young Farmers' Club have been motivated to participate in many practical ways. At the local level Heartbeat Wales has also been able to provide resources so that community projects for health have been established which draw on the lay organisations within that population. These have included community education classes on such diverse subjects as first-aid techniques and food preparation skills as well as the establishment of self-help groups for weight loss and those wishing to stop smoking.

Diffusion of innovations

The theory of diffusion of innovations (Rogers, 1983) explains how new attitudes, behaviours and products permeate and *spill* through social groups. It is clear that the adoption of lifestyles necessary to reduce the risks of heart disease can be speeded up by the actions and example of key opinion leaders within local communities. The use of exemplars was central to both the North Karelia and Stanford programmes. Consequently, establishing contact with both professional and lay opinion leaders has been a major activity for the Welsh Heart Programme Directorate. Groups have included GPs, community leaders, headteachers and journalists. The hope is that these key opinion leaders will not only encourage individuals to change through personal example, but will also accelerate the process by providing greater personal support and resources for health promotion.

Social marketing

The application of marketing principles to social change is known as social marketing (Fine, 1981; Kotler and Zaltman, 1971; Manoss, 1985). In particular, the Stanford project has studied this approach and has provided many good practical examples of its ability to reach individuals within a comprehensive programme (Maccoby and Alexander, 1980). The use of the media can be particularly effective in raising awareness and creating the right climate of opinion for change. Techniques of mass communication have already been used to good effect within the Welsh Heart Programme. At first this consisted of creating a national identity for the programme, establishing a corporate image — 'Heartbeat Wales' — and raising awareness of the problem and the need for action. As the programme became established, the media have been used as a trigger for action (for example, a television series was used to recruit people to first-aid training classes), or to support more personal approaches to health education (for example, special health kits have been recommended to help people lose weight, follow a healthier diet, and give up smoking).

Organisational change

Organisational change involves creating physical, social and economic environments which are beneficial to health. Health promotion programmes need to focus not only on the individual, but also on these external influences that shape lifestyles. A substantial part of the central initiative of Heartbeat Wales has been devoted to improving the 'macro-environment', which influences individual choice and opportunities for change (Parish, Caford and Honson, 1987). Examples in the area of nutrition include working with:

1. Farmers, purchasing specialists, and meat and milk marketing boards, in order to improve the nutritional content of food through better specifications, classifications and incentive schemes.
2. The food retail industry and supermarkets, to ensure that healthy foods are more widely available, appropriately labelled and sold at a price that Welsh people can afford.
3. Caterers in schools, workplaces and restaurants, in order to create better opportunities for healthy eating outside the home.

Given the differences in size and per capita budget between the Welsh Heart Programme and other international heart health projects these macro level initiatives have been uniquely important for the Welsh initiative and form a special component of the intervention.

Choice–Change–Champion Process

Research shows that behaviour change is initiated by exposure to powerful exemplars. The change will continue provided it is subsequently reinforced in an appropriate environment. An idealised sequence of events known as the Choice–Change–Champion process has been constructed by the authors to guide planning and priority setting. This model, presented in Figure 1, can be applied equally to the process of achieving change in individuals, groups and organisations (Catford, Nutbeam and Parish, 1987).

For effective intervention at community level three stages are required. The first concerns choice of a particular action — the *will* for change. The second concerns the actual change itself and its successful attainment — the *skill* for change. The final stage concerns the individual, group or organisation now acting as a change agent and becoming, a 'champion' for health — the *spill* for change. The process described below is at the level of the individual. It should be emphasised that it is not always necessary to follow the sequence precisely. However, each step has a unique contribution to make.

Choice

First, *awareness* about a particular health issue needs to be established. For example, it might be demonstrated that heart disease has reached epidemic proportions in the UK and that this is not improving as it is in other countries.

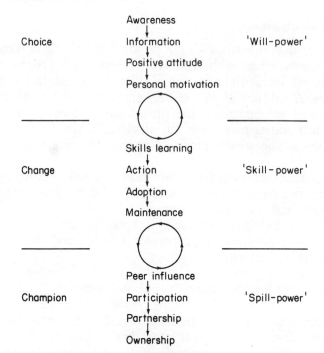

Figure 1   The Choice–Change–Champion process for health promotion.

Awareness can be increased through personal experience, mass communication and one-to-one education.

Information then needs to be provided by mass communication and one-to-one education. To continue with the above example, it would mean offering the information that a person can reduce this risk of a heart attack by not smoking, following a sensible diet and taking appropriate exercise.

A *positive attitude* then needs to be fostered. For example, it might be argued that non-smoking is the preferred health behaviour. An appropriate positive attitude can be created by promoting self-esteem, presenting attractive social modelling, using the influence of opinion leaders in the innovation-diffusion process, and through peer pressure.

Personal motivation is then required — for instance, to stop smoking. There is clear distinction between having a positive attitude to non-smoking, and internalising the belief 'I need and want to stop smoking'. Effective motivation requires setting short-term goals with positive incentives, with the lowest possible drawbacks. Another important factor is feedback.

Change

If action is to be successful, *skills training* needs to be provided. It is necessary to teach coping strategies; for example, would-be ex-smokers need to know how to handle cravings and possible weight increase, how to plan for cessation, and what to expect in general. They need to feel confident that they have every possibility of succeeding. Feelings of self-empowerment can be built up by providing further information but also through experience — for example, meeting successful ex-smokers and talking about their strategies. This area of skill-power is much undervalued by health professionals and is most necessary for those who find it difficult to change.

Action should then follow. This can often be triggered by cues; for example, an increase in the price of cigarettes, personal illness, pregnancy, or 'instructional' advice from a respected lay or professional person can be an important starting point. One approach currently being pursued with some success in Stanford and Minnesota involves contests — whereby successful quitters enter a lottery to win an attractive prize such as a holiday in Miami. Heartbeat Wales is using a similar approach as part of its exercise programme and in 1987 is launching a Heartbeat Exercise Contest open to all Welsh people aged 12–64.

Adoption then needs to be achieved. Many smokers require short-term support from lay or professional people. Nicorette chewing-gum and self-help groups may be helpful for some smokers. There also needs to be a supportive socioeconomic and physical environment conducive to non-smoking. For example, it may be possible to increase the availability of non-smoking areas in public places.

A programme of *maintenance* is also required. More than half the smokers who try to stop fail at their first attempt, but the more attempts they make the greater the likelihood of success. Positive reinforcements to maintain the change can be provided. For example, the social, interpersonal and financial rewards might be emphasised, so demonstrating the physical and symbolic benefits, and highlighting a sense of accomplishment.

Champion

In the past, many education programmes have gone no further than this — but those who have changed their lifestyles should be encouraged to move from the role of recipient to that of provider, from audience to actor.

First, converts can exert *peer influence* by accepting their roles as new opinion leaders. The next step from this is *participation*. Ex-smokers could, for example, give feedback to those planning smoking programmes. They could also press for environmental improvements for the non-smoking majority.

To increase their influence, such individuals might also take part in decision making about local programmes. Through the process of *partnership* they can assist in the planning, implementation and evaluation of community-based initiatives. However, the ultimate step is one of *ownership*, whereby lay people in a community become co-owners of health promotion initiatives and determine the future direction of programmes.

The challenge for the Welsh Heart Programme has been to refine, develop and implement this approach in a way appropriate to the unique social, cultural, economic and political situation in Wales. This process has already begun on two different fronts: in the local communities local opinion is sought and acted on, and at the national level there are discussions with the media, the food industry, government and major employers across Wales.

The following sections outline examples of practical action that have occurred since the inception of the Welsh Heart Programme.

Public Affairs and Mass Communication

The creation of a climate of opinion and interest conducive to the development of the programme was a major goal during the first 12 months. Mass communication techniques can be used effectively to convey simple messages to large numbers of people at a relatively low cost. Approximately one-sixth of the first year's budget was used to finance media activities. The printed and broadcast media were both employed extensively, the main aims being to raise awareness about the need for community action and to enlist the support of the public, the professionals and politicians. The Welsh language is used extensively in certain parts of Wales, so a bilingual policy was adopted at the outset.

It was also decided that advertising time and space should not be purchased. The programme would be newsworthy in itself if it was succeeding in its goal of community involvement. In the event, extensive coverage was provided by the local and regional press, local radio, and national and regional television. The mass media activities during 1985 culminated in an extremely successful six-part television series on BBC Wales entitled 'Don't Break Your Heart'. The series examined lifestyles and was shown during peak viewing time. The series was co-produced by Heartbeat Wales. In addition, Heartbeat Wales has collaborated with independent television and the BBC in the production of a number of other health related television programmes, namely; 'Go for it', 'You are what you Eat', 'Broken Hearts' and, in Wales, 'A Stake in your Heart'. Assistance has also been provided for the television broadcasts associated with the 'Save a Life' campaign — which aims at enabling as many lay people as possible to acquire the ability to provide first aid for heart attack victims.

In addition to the news coverage and editorial comment generated by the programme's activities, Heartbeat Wales also produced three issues of a 12-page newspaper that was distributed as an insert in the major regional press. By the third issue, the newspaper had achieved a circulation of 300,000 and had a potential readership approaching one million; which is one third of the population of Wales.

Wales is a nation with a strong tradition of county shows and events, particularly during the summer period. As part of the process of raising awareness and community involvement, Heartbeat Wales, in conjunction with the health authorities, had a presence at most of the major county and agricultural shows during 1985 and 1986. The exhibition work will continue throughout the initial five-year lifetime of the project, albeit at a reduced level of activity. This work has been considerably assisted by the recent donation of six pantechnicon trailers, which have been converted with the help of the

Manpower Services Commission. Five of these vehicles, provided by Tesco, the leading supermarket chain in Wales, have been made available to health authorities for use as mobile exhibition and lifestyle appraisal units.

Co-operation with television continued during 1986 with two co-produced ten-part series about healthy eating being broadcast on S4C and HTV from October into December. Information packs and health kits were produced to support the television broadcasts. The programmes appear to have been popular, since some 200,000 packs and kits have been distributed to date. By the mid-point of the HTV series, 37 per cent of Welsh people had watched at least one programme. The overall success of the high media profile is illustrated by a survey conducted one year after the launch of the programme. This showed that 53 per cent of the Welsh population were aware of Heartbeat Wales and 97 per cent considered it a worthwhile enterprise (WHPD, 1986b). This had risen to 68 per cent by March 1988 (Beaufort Research Welsh Omnibus Series, 1988).

The original 1984 planning document prepared by the Health Education Council envisaged that approximately one-third of the programme's budget would be spent on mass media initiatives, but the success in generating media interest has meant that this figure has been reduced. There is little doubt that mass communication methods will continue to play an important role during the remainder of the programme. The mass media can provide an avenue for raising public awareness and transmitting simple messages. They also have a role in the teaching of limited skills (for example, cooking techniques) and can provide cues for action. Without doubt the media can assist in creating a social climate conducive to change, but the power of the mass media alone to change behaviour should not be over-rated. It is in conjunction with other more personal approaches that media techniques will be most effective.

Health Authorities

The importance of the nine health authorities in the Principality was recognised at the outset. Action at the local level might have been seriously hampered without their participation. Key personnel in each authority were contacted at the outset of the programme and the authorities were asked to consider undertaking three specific roles. First, to provide general support for activities generated at the national level. Second, each authority was asked to monitor and co-ordinate action within their specific county. Finally, each was asked to identify two or three local priorities for possible financial support from Heartbeat Wales, the intention being to establish a network of local pilot projects covering the range of activities described in the consultative document *Take Heart*.

In order to assist this process, each authority was asked to establish a multi-disciplinary planning group. Although health education departments undertook the responsibility for much of the work involved in planning and co-ordination, the response from health authorities in general was excellent and the programme could not have progressed so rapidly without their support. Each authority has at least one CHD Planning Group in operation and some of these have broadened their remit to embrace other health promotion and prevention issues.

Advice and support was provided for by the development of district smoking, and food and health policies. Most of the authorities had already made inroads on the smoking issue prior to the advent of the Welsh Heart Programme and two had started to develop food and health policies. All the authorities now have smoking and diet programmes, at least in the late planning stages, and most are in the process of implementation.

The ambulance services have also lent considerable support to the programme by actively promoting educational schemes to teach cardiopulmonary resuscitation (CPR) skills to the public and by carrying advertising on the side of their vehicles. A national programme under the banner of 'Heartstart Wales' is now underway as part of the 'Save a Life' campaign and in many areas the voluntary ambulance services are also involved.

In addition to smoking, diet and CPR, health and local Authorities are being encouraged to develop co-ordinated programmes for blood pressure screening and control, and for the promotion of sensible forms of aerobic exercise.

Heartbeat Wales has allocated almost a third of its budget over the period 1986 to 1989 to support local initiatives. This recognises the fact that it would be unreasonable for hard-pressed health authorities and their health education units to undertake a considerable increase in workload without a corresponding increase in resources. However, authorities were advised early in the planning process that financial support would not be available unless additional funds were also generated at the local level on a roughly matched basis. Heartbeat Wales did not insist that such funds should be allocated from the health authority's budget; indeed, it was suggested that other agencies, such as the Manpower Services Commission, family practitioner committees, and county and borough councils, might also lend their support for community projects.

Voluntary subscription and commercial sponsorship were also suggested as potentially advantageous avenues to explore. Despite some initial resistance to the idea of local funding, arrangements were made with all the authorities and a total sum in excess of £400,000 was channelled into local programmes during 1987/1988. Most of the activities described in *Take Heart* will be undertaken by one or more local programmes, and all were operational by February 1987.

Primary Health Care

Heartbeat Wales supports the proposals for the prevention of cardiovascular disease outlined in a report by the Welsh Council of the Royal College of General Practitioners (RCGP, 1983). This report recommended routine recording of smoking and blood pressure, as well as opportunistic health education about diet and general fitness. The moves towards increased anticipatory care were assisted during 1987 by the appointment of a number of primary care facilitators as part of the local programmes mentioned above. Some of these facilitators will operate along the lines of the Oxford Heart Attack and Stroke Project (Fullard, Fowler and Gray 1984; also see elsewhere in this collection), although it is also the intention to experiment with alternative models of support.

The Welsh Council's report also stressed the importance of appropriate education for all members of the primary health care team. Heartbeat Wales has collaborated closely with the Open University in the development of a distance learning course on cardiovascular disease prevention for primary health care practitioners. The course is entitled *Reducing the Risk* (Open University, 1987). This has been promoted extensively in Wales since it became available in March 1987 and is now used more widely than anywhere else in the UK.

Heartbeat Wales is also funding a pilot project designed to enhance the health education skills of pharmacists and dentists. Another pilot scheme organised by the Mid Glamorgan Health Authority and the Nursing Department of the University of Wales College of Medicine is currently being funded by Heartbeat Wales. This scheme is to assess the potential role of the health visitor in promoting family health.

Schools and Young People

During 1986 a major survey was undertaken in Welsh secondary schools (WHPD, 1986c) to determine knowledge, attitudes and behaviour in relation to a number of lifestyle issues. The information arising from this is assisting in the planning of a Welsh Youth Health Programme. Research on the nature and extent of health education in Welsh schools has also recently been completed and this, combined with the health survey of young people, provides a unique and comprehensive information base for further developments.

Considerable curriculum development work has been carried out by the Health Education Council in recent years. Rather than duplicate this effort, Heartbeat Wales has been promoting existing curriculum projects where appropriate. A decision was taken early in the programme to concentrate attention on the 9–13 age group, since it is at this age that many young people start to acquire a greater degree of independence, and begin to experiment with unhealthy behaviour patterns that may be carried through into adult life.

The school system enables the most ready access to young people. The 'My Body' Project is a well-evaluated curriculum package that has been shown to reduce smoking experimentation (Murray *et al.*, 1982). Heartbeat Wales, in conjunction with health education departments, has promoted this project in primary schools and will be providing support through a continuing programme of in-service training for teachers. 'My Body' focuses on the functioning of the heart and lungs, and is particularly relevant to smoking education. Additional modules on nutrition and exercise have been commissioned as part of the development of the programme.

A health club has been established for children of primary school age, initially on a pilot basis, in Pembrokeshire and thus has now been extended to two other counties. The main intention of this club is to involve children, outside the curriculum, in issues concerning their health and that of their community. Members, known as 'Heartguards', receive a regular newsletter and participate in competitions and quizzes.

Local Authorities

There are 37 local councils in Wales and much of the work that has been undertaken to date has been in collaboration with their Environmental Health Departments. In January 1986 Heartbeat Wales launched a pilot project with four environmental health departments to promote non-smoking areas and improve menu choices within eating establishments. The scheme, administered by environmental health officers as part of their routine food hygiene inspections, involved the provision of a 'Heartbeat Award' to any establishment conforming to a set of specific criteria. Twenty-five councils have now agreed to join the scheme and awards have been given to a large number of restaurants, hotels, schools, hospitals, fast food outlets and public houses.

Local councils and Heartbeat Wales have also collaborated in building a number of exercise circuits and walks in pleasant countryside or parks. These 'Heartbeat Ways' and 'Heartbeat Walks' have been designed with graded levels of activity to enable people of any age, fitness or ability to participate.

The Workplace

The workplace provides an opportunity to take elements of the programme to large numbers of people who share a common environment for much of the day. Many of the larger employers provide occupational health services and there has been considerable interest amongst managers, unions and occupational health staff in plans to develop screening and general health promotion activities for the workforce. A number of programmes have been initiated with major employers, including British Airways, Ford and the National Coal Board. The Wales TUC has agreed a joint policy statement with Heartbeat Wales on promoting health in the workplace and 18,000 copies of this have been made available throughout Wales. In the summer of 1988 Heartbeat Wales, in partnership with the CBI, launched a prestigious award called 'Health is your Business' designed to encourage employers to support health initiatives in the workplace.

Conclusions

The experience of Heartbeat Wales shows that a health promotion campaign that aims to encourage participation at every level can be successful. Change is occurring throughout Wales at both community and organisational levels. There is every indication that health is improving. Three years after the programme was launched, a follow-up questionnaire survey of 1,000 adults was carried out in September 1988. This showed that large numbers of Welsh people were reporting important behavioural changes. Seven per cent had stopped smoking for more than 3 months in the last year and a quarter of current smokers were trying to give up at the time of the survey. Over a third (39 per cent) of all adults reported to having consciously changed their diet to a healthier one. Twenty-six per cent had successfully lost more than 5 lbs in weight in the last year and twenty per cent reported increasing their level of exercise by at least 60 minutes per week. Fifty-three per cent had had their blood pressure checked in the past year. The changes were observed in both sexes, all ages and social groups, and throughout the whole of Wales. In addition over a third (35 per cent) of the adult population in Wales reported that they had changed their diet to a healthier one. Over a quarter (28 per cent) had successfully lost more than five pounds in weight in the last year. Many (28 per cent) also said that they were taking more regular exercise, and over a half (54 per cent) of those questioned had presented to have their blood pressure checked in the past year. The changes were observed in both sexes, all ages and social groups, and throughout the whole of Wales.

If these improvements in lifestyle are confirmed by follow-up studies and can be maintained over time, the prospects for better health in Wales are most encouraging.

References and Bibliography

Bandura, A. (1977) *Social Learning Theory*. Prentice Hall, Englewood Cliffs, NJ.

Blackburn, H. (1983) 'Research and Demonstration Projects in Community Cardiovascular Disease Prevention', *Journal of Public Health Policy*, **4**, 4.

Blackburn, H., Luepker, R., Kline, F., Bracht, N., Carlow, R., Jacobs, D., Mittelmark, M., Stauffer, L., Taylor, H. (1984) 'The Minnesota Heart Health Programme: a Research and Development Project in Cardiovascular Disease Prevention', in Mattarazzo, J., Weiss, S., Herd, J. *et al.* (eds) *Behavioural Health: A Handbook of Health Enhancement and Disease Prevention*. John Wiley, New York.

Bracht, N., Mittelmark, M., Luepker, R. (1987) 'Community Analysis Precedes Community Organisation for Cardiovascular Disease Prevention: The Minnesota Heart Health Programme', Division of Epidemiology, University of Minnesota (Submitted for publication).

Catford, J. C., Nutbeam, D., Parish, R. (1987) 'Promoting Health in the Community: The Choice-Change-Champion Process' (Submitted for publication).

Department of Health and Social Security (1984) *Diet and Cardiovascular Disease*, Report of the Committee on Medical Aspects of Food Policy (COMA). HMSO, London.

Farquhar, J. W. (1978) 'The Community Based Model of Lifestyle Intervention Trials', *American Journal of Epidemiology*, **108**, 103–111.

Farquhar, J. W., Fortman, S. P., Wood, P. D. (1983) 'Community Studies of Cardiovascular Disease Prevention', in Kaplan, N. M. and Stamler, J. (eds) *Prevention of Coronary Heart Disease: Practical Management of Risk Factors*. W. B. Saunders, Eastbourne.

Farquhar, J., Fortmann, S., Maccoby, N., Wood, P., Haskell, W., Barr Taylor, C., Flora, J., Solomon, D., Rogers, T., Adler, E., Breitrose, P., Weiner, L. (1984) 'The Stanford Five City Project: an Overview', in Matarazzo, J., Weiss, S., Herd, J. *et al.* (eds) *Behavioural Health: A Handbook of Health Enhancement and Disease Prevention*. John Wiley, New York.

Farquhar, J. W., Fortman, S. P., Maccoby, N. (1984) *The Stanford Five City Project: Design and Methods*. Stanford Heart Disease Prevention Programme, Stanford University School of Medicine, Stanford.

Fine, S. H. (1981) *The Marketing of Ideas and Social Issues*. Praeger, New York.

Fullard, E., Fowler, G., and Gray, M. (1984) 'Facilitating Prevention in Primary Care'. *British Medical Journal*, **289**, 1585–1587.

Jacobs, D. R., Luepker, R. V., Mittelmark, M. (1985) 'Community Wide Prevention Strategies: Evaluation Design of the Minnesota Heart Health Programme', *Journal of Chronic Diseases*.

Kotler, P., and Zaltman, G. (1971) 'Social Marketing: An Approach to Plan social change', *Journal of Marketing*, **35**, 3–12.

Lasater, T., Abrams, D., Artz, L., Beaudin, P., Cabrera, L., Elder, J., Ferreira, A., Kinsley, P., Peterson, G., Rodrigues, A., Rosenberg, P., Snow, R., Carleton, R. (1984) 'Lay Volunteer Delivery of a, Community Based Cardiovascular Risk Factor Change Programme: the Pawtucket Experiment, in Matarazzo. J., Weiss, S., Herd, J. *et al.* (eds) *Behavioural Health: A Handbook of Health Enhancement and Disease Prevention*. John Wiley, New York.

Maccoby, N., Farquhar, J., Wood, P., Alexander, J. (1977) 'Reducing the Risk of Cardiovascular Disease: Effects of a Community Based Campaign on Knowledge and Behaviour', *Journal of Community Health*, **3**, 100–114.

Maccoby, N., and Alexander, J. (1980) 'Use of Media in Lifestyle Programmes', in Davidson, P. O. (ed.) *Behavioural Medicine: Changing Health Lifestyles*. Bruner Mazel, New York.

Manoss, R. K. (1985) *Social Marketing New Imperative for Public Health*. Praeger, New York.

Murray, M., Swan, A.V., Enoch, C., Johnson, M.R.D., Banks, M.H., Reid, D.J. (1982) 'The Effectiveness of the Health Education Council's "My Body' School Education Project', *Health Education Journal*, **41**, 126–130.

Nutbeam, D., and Catford, J. (1987) 'Welsh Heart Programme Evaluation Strategy. Progress, Plans and Possibilities', *Health Promotion*, Vol No. 2.

Open University (1987) *Coronary Heart Disease — Reducing the Risks*, Course P575. Open University Press, Milton Keynes.

Parish, R., Catford, J., and Howson, H. (1987) 'Promoting Health through Collaboration with Commerce and Industry — Experience of the Welsh Heart Programme', in *Community Based Prevention and Health Promotion — Report of an International Conference*. German Society of Social and Prophylactic Medicine, and WHO, Dusseldorf.

Parish, R., Catford, J., Nutbeam, D. (1987). Breathing Life into Wales: Progress of the Welsh Heart Programme. *Health Trends*. **19**.

Puska, P., Nissinen, A., Salonen, J. T., Tuomilehto, J., Koskela, K., McAlister, A., Kottke, T., Maccoby, N., Farquhar, J. (1985) 'The Community Based Strategy to Prevent Coronary Heart Disease: Conclusions from the Ten Years of the North Karelia Project', *Annual Reviews of Public Health*.

Rogers, E., and Kuncaid, D. (1981) *Communication Networks: Toward a New Paradigm for Research*. The Free Press, New York.

Rogers, E. (1983) *Diffusion of Innovations*. The Free Press/Macmillan, London.

Rose, G., Ball, K., Catford, J. (1984) *Coronary Heart Disease Prevention: Plans for Action*. Pitman, London.

Royal College of General Practitioners (Welsh Council) (1983) *Stitches in Time — Proposals for Action on the Prevention of Coronary Heart Disease and Stroke by General Practitioners in Wales*. Royal College of General Practitioners, London.

Tuomilehto, J., Nuttaanmaki, L., Salonen, J., Puska, P., Nissinen, A. (1983) 'Community Involvement in Developing Comprehensive Cardiovascular Control programmes: a case study in North Karelia, Finland' *Yearbook of Population Research in Finland*, XXI/1983. Population Research Institute, Helsinki.

Welsh Heart Programme Directorate (1985). *Take Heart: A Consultative Document on the Development of Community-based Heart Health Initiatives within Wales.* Heartbeat Report No. 1, WHP, 24 Park Place, Cardiff, UK.

Welsh Heart Programme Directorate (1986a) *Pulse of Wales: Preliminary Report of the Welsh Heart Health Survey 1985.* Heartbeat Report No. 4, WHP, 24 Park Place, Cardiff, UK.

Welsh Heart Programme Directorate (1986b). *Heartbeat Wales Awareness and Recall Survey Report.* Heartbeat Report No. 6, WHP, 24 Park Place, Cardiff, UK.

Welsh Heart Programme Directorate (1986c) *Welsh Youth Health Survey Protocol.* Heartbeat Report No. 5, WHP, 24 Park Place, Cardiff, UK.

Welsh Heart Programme Directorate (1986d) *Smoking or Youth. Reducing Teenage Smoking in Wales.* Heartbeat Report No. 8, WHP, 24 Park Place, Cardiff, UK.

World Health Organization (1978). *Primary Health Care. Report of the International Conference on Primary Health Care.* Alma-Ata, USSR, 6–12 September 1978. WHO, Geneva.

World Health Organization (1982) *Prevention of Coronary Heart Disease.* Report of a WHO Expert Committee, Technical Report Series No. 678, WHO, Geneva.

World Health Organization (1984) *Health Promotion: A Discussion Document on the Concept and Principles.* WHO (Euro), Copenhagen.

World Health Organization (1986) *Community Prevention and Control of Cardiovascular Diseases.* Report of a WHO Expert Committee; Technical Report Series No. 732, WHO, Geneva.

World Health Organization (1987) *Ottawa Charter for Health Promotion.* Presented by the First International Conference on Health Promotion, 21 November 1986. WHO (Euro), Copenhagen.

Welsh Omnibus Survey (1988) Prepared for Welsh Health Promotion Authority. March 1988.

Changing Ideas in Health Care
Edited by D. Seedhouse and A. Cribb
© 1989 John Wiley & Sons Ltd

Chapter Eight
'Powell Street': Community Mental Health

KAREN NEWBIGGING, TONY CADMAN AND JUNE WESTLEY
Community Mental Health Service
Manchester
UK

Introduction

There is a growing discussion among people working in the human services about the principles and values upon which services for people are based. Grounded in the recognition that all services provided to people are value-based, many plans and policies now start by making these values explicit, usually as a set of statements of belief about the rights of the client group concerned (Malin, 1987). 'Powell Street' is an early example of a community mental health service that used this approach to planning. The result of a commitment to involve the local community in the process, and to incorporate information about the community's skills and resources into the planning, was the emergence of a new kind of mental health service.

This chapter aims to describe this process, to reflect some of the experiences of the service and to highlight some of the themes relevant to the rapid development of community mental health services in this country.

Planning for People

In north Manchester in the early 1980s most existing facilities for people with mental health problems were organised on the site of the District General Hospital, part of which was founded in the late nineteenth century and used as a workhouse. It now serves as the in-patient facility, has three day hospitals, and is the site for out-patient appointments for people with mental health problems. There was concern about the accessibility of these services to people living in the south-east of the health district, since they faced a long journey to the hospital. There was also anxiety that the nature of these facilities increased the stigma of having a mental health problem. The community physician, Dr Judith Gray, was asked to evaluate the possibility of establishing a day centre in that part of the health district. Dr Gray wanted to avoid what she saw as the usual health service approach to planning, which was to start with a building and create a service to fit it (Gray, 1985). The planning process therefore aimed to:

1. Look afresh at the needs of people.
2. Propose a service that would avoid the depersonalisation that often accompanies services and institutions.
3. Propose a service that would not only help to relieve the immediate problems of people, but also contribute to identifying and altering the factors contributing to the development of problems.
4. Propose a service that would keep clients in the community and not compound their difficulties by stigmatising them.
5. Propose a service that would encourage relationships outside those with other clients and professionals.
6. Propose a service suited to the needs of people living in a locality that is amongst the most disadvantaged in an inner city health district, having few resources in terms of leisure, employment and housing.

(Openshaw Outreach Mental Health Project, 1984)

A whole range of people were involved, including psychiatrists, psychologists, nurses, representatives of social services and a church minister from the local community. In order that the future service should meet the *real* needs of clients, the planning process began by looking at the lives of people who were using existing facilities at the general hospital, or at the local health centre. This approach to planning was derived from PASS (Programme Analysis of Service Systems), an instrument originally developed to plan and evaluate services for people with learning difficulties. PASS is based on the principle of normalisation (Wolfensberger, 1972), which starts with the premise that all people are valued citizens of equal status, regardless of their disability. Services are often planned on the basis of people's disabilities rather than their abilities or needs. The principle of normalisation argues that the goal of services should be to support someone with a disability in such a way that he or she can live within the local community and participate in that community as a valued member (Brost, *et al.*, 1982). In using this theory to plan a local community health service, it was hoped that the autonomy and independence of a person would be encouraged, and the isolation that occurs with people who become long-term users of psychiatric services could be avoided.

In order to understand the needs of people currently using mental health services, for whom the service was being planned, members of the planning body spent time with people building up a picture of their lives and histories. The members looked at what this group of people had in common with other people and what was different about them. From listening, going to therapy sessions, asking them about their interests and their past, eating the same meals, and meeting their friends, a number of themes emerged:

1. There was very little opportunity for people using mental health services to work and play among different types of people.

2. People had few possessions.
3. People often had no sense of autonomy or individuality.
4. There was little opportunity to make relationships or to meet people who were not either mentally ill or staff of mental illness services.
5. People had little continuity in terms of either the staff looking after them or the places they were in.

(Gray, 1985)

The next step (see Figure 1) was to look at the sorts of skills and resources that might be needed to fulfil evident needs, and then to compare these with existing skills in order to identify what extra skills might be necessary. A research assistant worked voluntarily to build up a profile of the local area. His task was to examine the strengths and weaknesses of the local community, its resources, and its social composition.

> It [the community] could be hostile, unhelpful, dangerous and lacking in resources and knowledge. None the less it was important to have information, to build participation and to find ways to empower the community rather than to manipulate and exploit it. We tried to see our task as service developers as integration — coordinating and linking as far as possible the needs and strengths of the individual with what was already (and potentially) there in the community.

(Gray, 1985)

From this work it was possible to propose the types of extra resources required. Basically these were ordinary community resources, such as cafes and clubs where people could meet, places to teach practical skills, give advice, and support; places where people could feel safe and where voluntary and self-help groups could meet. Within these resources workers would offer individual people support, not only in dealing with their immediate problems, but also in leading a more fulfilling life. They would also support self-help groups and

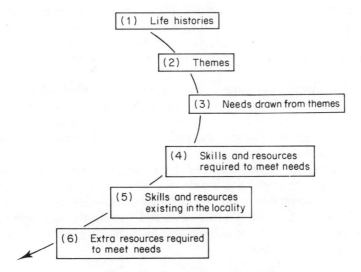

Figure 1 Approach to planning.

develop training for other people to enable them to help someone with mental health problems. The workers would assist in the use and development of community resources and in particular it was proposed that someone would liaise with and learn about the people (and other resources) in the area, as well as encouraging the growth of new resources.

It was proposed that the service would not stigmatise and although it would have a physical base in the locality, it would, wherever possible, attempt to work with people in their everyday environments. There would be consumer, family and community involvement in planning and review of the service, and in therapy and evaluation. In addition, a commitment to evaluation was stated.

It was hoped by using this approach of working with people within their everyday settings, and by offering support at an earlier stage in the development of mental health problems, that the autonomy and independence of people would be encouraged, and the marginalisation that exists when people became long-term users of psychiatric services could be avoided.

'POWELL STREET'

Description of the service

1985 saw the plans become reality, when a team of five people was employed to develop the proposed service. The team (clinical psychologist, community nurse therapist, social worker, receptionist and community mental health worker) employed by Health and Social Services, are based in a terraced house, No. 2 Powell Street, in an inner city area that is predominantly working class.

The service has four main aims:

1. To provide a local mental health service to the residents of a defined inner city area, a population of about 25,000.
2. To reintegrate users of the service within their local community.
3. To work towards changing public attitudes to mental illness.
4. To work with others in the locality to help the community develop its own resources and encourage people to make good use of these resources.

By and large, word of mouth has proved the most effective form of communication about Powell Street, although other ways of publicising the service have been tried. These have included the circulation of posters, newsheets and leaflets to statutory and voluntary agencies and information centres. Articles in the local newspaper and interviews on the radio have stimulated interest, although usually from outside the area. Meeting local groups and talking briefly about the service was one of the main ways in which the team and local people tried to publicise Powell Street in its early days. For example, going to a local social club and having the microphone for five minutes before the call for 'eyes down and look in' signalled the start of bingo, was one novel avenue tried.

The public meetings and extensive discussions that had taken place during the planning stages to inform and involve the local community were also helpful. A number of meetings were held once the workers were employed and an emphasis developed on using social occasions as a way of advertising the service. For instance, prior to the house being open for callers, 150 households in the immediate neighbourhood were invited to come to see the house and meet the team. Although only 35 people accepted this invitation it was a good start to getting known.

Physical base

The location and type of building in which the service is housed has been enormously helpful in shaping its development. The house itself is at an end of a terrace and therefore slightly larger than other houses in the street. Apart from this it looks similar to the other houses. It is distinguished only by a large number '2' over the porch. This similarity and the absence of labels causes most professionals to comment on the difficulty they have locating it, though few local people have such difficulty. In addition to not being obviously different, the fact that the house was previously used as a home and has no historical associations with 'devaluing images', is also important. In the downstairs part of the house there is a reception area, a room large enough for group discussions, and a kitchen for people to 'brew up'. Upstairs there are two offices, an interview room and a room used by community groups.

This style of accommodation lends itself to the development of a service that is more informal and offers a comfortable atmosphere for people using the service. Organising a service in this way does not automatically solve all the problems inherent in using psychiatric services, but it makes it more likely that people using the service are not so stigmatised, increases the opportunities for the service and its consumers to be seen as part of the local community, and means that staff are more accessible to local people and therefore likely to be more responsive.

Although the building does provide a focus for the service it has never been the intention that all the work should take place within its four walls. There has always been an emphasis on using other local settings, from people's homes, church halls and GP's surgeries to local schools and community centres. These other settings are more likely to be used for meetings, courses and social gatherings, whilst the house is the place where people know they can contact the workers or use the other resources available. In order to be able to develop work outside this base, formal open hours are restricted to three times a week for people to drop-in, but in practice there are many callers outside these times.

Importantly, the house also provides a place for other people to meet. One of the rooms is used regularly by the local residents and consumers who form the Community Planning Group. A self-help group, 'People against Depression', also use the building one or two evenings a week, and it is used by other groups such as MIND and a community drugs team from time to time.

A Better Mental Health Service

The team's aim in providing a mental health service is to help people develop their skills and confidence so that they are able to identify and tackle their problems and develop more satisfying lifestyles. In parallel with this we encourage people to move away from viewing themselves as 'ill', where their needs might best be met by medical responses, to a position where they have a broader insight into life, its problems and the resources that can be mobilised to tackle those problems. Helping someone to develop their self-confidence, and improve the ways in which they engage with the social world, is a process that takes place at three different levels at Powell Street. These are the individual, group and community levels.

1. At the level of the individual

Referral   Powell Street has an open referral system, which means that anyone can refer to the service. Families, neighbours, social workers, general practitioners, consultant psychiatrists, and the individuals themselves refer. Indeed we have found that the highest proportion of referrals is made up of people who refer themselves. Referrals are made by telephone, letter or in person, although it is the last of these that is encouraged. The drop-in times offer an opportunity for people to come and meet at least two of the workers, find out about the service, and discuss the sort of help they are seeking. One of the workers is also available on a regular basis at a local GP's surgery.

MIND, following a visit in 1986 to Powell Street, observed that:

> . . . of the users we talked with, two had been referred to Powell Street by a social worker or a psychiatrist. The others' initial contact with the service indicates a degree of success in establishing an accessible service with good links locally: one person had been recommended both by a psychiatrist and by neighbours, and one heard of Powell Street when two of the staff gave a talk at a local community education centre and one just walked in, after seeing a leaflet in the Post Office.

First contact   People's first experiences of contact with a service are important. If people call we try to make them feel welcome and try to find out a bit about them. We give information about our service, who works there and what is on offer, so that people have some basis on which to decide whether they would like to participate. This can be a difficult balance to achieve since it is important to help people feel at ease and in control of the situation rather than being overwhelmed by information. People come with a range of requests, or are referred for different reasons. Some people know exactly what help they want whereas others, as is more often the case, come feeling upset or dissatisfied with their lives. The task is then to begin to help the person articulate what the problem is and how he or she might begin to tackle it. Looking at people who come to Powell Street it is possible to characterise their difficulties in broad terms, as illustrated in Table 1. Any categorisation of problems is unsatisfactory since people rarely have neatly defined problems and may be experiencing difficulties in a number of areas. Sometimes people ask for specific information, but more usually they have persisting difficulties. Roughly three-quarters of the people we meet have had extensive and sometimes unsatisfying experiences with other mental health services.

Table 1 Request for personal support

Problem category	Examples
Personal distress grief, depression, anxiety, stress, physical symptoms	A woman referred herself because she was extremely disabled by panic attacks
	A young man experiencing visual hallucinations referred by his GP
Family problems marital conflict, problems with children,	A couple referred by their GP as they are no longer able to talk to each other without arguing
caring for someone else such as an elderly relative	A man asked for help because he was finding the strain of caring for his wife, who was disabled, too much
	A local resident was worried about a neighbour, who was discovered to be in an acute psychotic state
Social isolation	A woman diagnosed as 'having schizophrenia', referred by a psychiatrist because she had become extremely isolated since the death of her mother
Lack of activity	A man being discharged from hospital, referred by social worker because he had nothing to occupy him
	Request for information about becoming a volunteer
Welfare housing, legal, financial and welfare rights	A mother of a son with 'schizophrenia' asked for help with a complex housing problem
	A young woman who had lost access to her children asking about her rights
Service inadequate coordination of services,	A man referred himself for help as he was in the process of being discharged from a psychiatric hospital and thought it was happening too quickly
dissatisfaction,	
request for information	Request for information about support groups for women following hysterectomy

Later contact   Working with individuals can involve:

practical help,
emotional support,
counselling,
building up specific skills, for example assertiveness,
access to information about what is on locally, often coupled with support
to get involved,
liaising with other statutory voluntary agencies and self-help groups.

In addition to working with the individuals themselves, their partners, their families and other members of their close community may also be involved.

Although requests for help are usually initiated on an individual basis it is often possible to involve someone in other aspects of the service, as well as or instead of offering support on a personal basis. People frequently move from using only personal support to participation in group or community activities.

2.   At the level of the group

As workers learn more about the people with whom they are working, they gain a better understanding of what those people's lives are really like. As this happens, opportunities arise to bring people together to discuss common concerns.

An example of the way this works in practice is the team's early response to the ways in which women and men were presenting to the service. In the first three months a striking pattern emerged and it was noticeable that over a third of all the women referred were aged between 40 and 50. For many of these women the difficulties they talked about reflected isolation, little to do, loss of a valued role through divorce or children leaving home, family difficulties and the menopause. The two women on the team, together with a community worker and a woman who had called at Powell Street with her social worker, decided to invite all the women to get together. Over 20 women accepted this invitation and came along to a meeting. This group of women split into smaller groups to discuss what they needed to change their lives (see Table 2).

From the discussion that followed, the women decided to set up a club with a strong social element that would be run by its members. It was intended to create an opportunity for support and to enable the development of confidence and social skills. The workers were to be used as a resource to draw on. This club has now been running for two and a half years and its members have done a range of different things — including swimming for the first time in years, setting up a stall on the local market to raise money, organising social evenings out, embarking on a holiday in the Lake District, and taking up yoga.

Perhaps the main benefit has been that the weekly meetings allow the women just to get together and chat. An important outcome of this club is the friendships that have developed. This has resulted in some of the women meeting to do things together outside the club. The number of women who

Table 2 Feedback from consulting women about what they need

Group 1
Support, company of women
Sense of identity
Time to be self/feminine
Social/outings
Using each others skills, e.g. hairdressing
Health—learning about it
Assertion group training

Group 2
Support group—women only
Confidence building
Group to go out in the evening
Company
Taster courses, e.g. maths
Crafts
Women's health sessions
Assertion training

Group 3
Being understood, support
Find own identity
Regain capabilities
Time for self, confidence
Liking myself again
Social life
Educational group-health
You can't talk the same with men

Group 4
Women's support
Be me! Finding out who me is–
   find out things that make you happy
Nights out, mixing, doing things together
Sharing experiences
Away from labels

now come to the club is small. This is a reflection of the success of the club since some women have left to do other things, including work, attending college and going on holiday. These are all activities that suggest a social role quite different from that which existed when their initial contact with Powell Street was made.

The other development to grow out of the women's club was an assertiveness course, run by the two women workers. The workers and the women felt that although the club provided good opportunities there was also a need to focus on problems and to develop skills and confidence for dealing with these, in order to strengthen the women's sense of identity.

The attention given to women raised the issue of gender differences in the use of mental health services. It begged the question about the relative under-use of the service by men and led us to consider their needs. In response to these concerns the two male workers took the initiative of developing a course on 'Men and Mental Health' to create a forum for men working locally to consider these issues.

Bringing people together is an important part of our work and other ways in which this has happened include:

(i) Initiating groups that meet regularly. An example One worker established a writers' group after several consumers had talked about how they would like to write. Previous unhappy experience of formal education, combined with current lifestyle, had restricted opportunities for these people to develop their creative potential. Not yet ready to participate in adult education, this group began by describing everyday situations. They have met other writers' groups and are currently writing a play — a skit on psychiatry — that they plan to read to both local and professional audiences.

Recognising that people have untapped potential prompted a health promotion officer to offer a creative therapy group for people involved with Powell Street. Other examples include establishing a carer's support group, to help develop a support network to mitigate the stress and isolation involved in being a carer. The stress of caring for someone else is now well documented (Finch and Groves, 1983), and it seemed to us that bringing people together was the most useful way of providing support.

(ii)   Inviting people to get together to consider an issue   Issues that have emerged for many people using the service include work, benefits, creche facilities and tranquilisers. In response to this we have invited people to get together so that they have an opportunity to consider possible ways forward. Typically this has involved outside agencies who have access to relevant information and resources.

(iii)   Running courses   The development of an educational programme has been another feature of the service. The aim of the courses provided has been to pass on skills, ideas and knowledge related to mental well-being. One example is the assertiveness course. Other examples include the 'Men and Mental Health' course, 'Caring for Carers', and a course on counselling skills. A health course, run at a local GP's surgery, was aimed at encouraging people to look at ways of being healthy in their own lives, and also at raising the awareness of mental health at that particular surgery. This approach subtly shifts the emphasis from the problems being seen as difficulties that are shared. In promoting an educational rather than a therapeutic response these difficulties are shown to be relevant to everyone.

3.   At the level of community work

The ways in which psychiatric services have traditionally been organised have compounded the difficulties facing someone experiencing mental ill-health. People using mental health services have been found to have not only fewer networks but also a poorer quality of relationships.

A key feature of service organisation has been the segregation of people with mental health problems in psychiatric hospitals, day hospitals, day centres, and industrial therapy centres. The only opportunities remaining for contact with other people in the same trap are those offered by meetings with paid staff and family. When the people planning Powell Street looked at the lives of people using services they found that these people shared a need for real and meaningful relationships on many different levels, and also needed a choice of things to do.

As well as working with individual people to achieve these aims, the community has been targeted as a focus for integration. At this level our work involves:

1. Developing local networks of care and support. For example, a local volunteer centre has been developed in conjunction with a local curate and the Council for Voluntary Service.
2. Developing relationships with local groups and people. Initially we saw this as a priority and have continued to make an input into various community organisations.
3. Using existing networks and organisations so that people with mental health difficulties are included and catered for within their programme and events.
4. Holding events to publicise the work of Powell Street and to draw people's attention to mental health issues. For example, open meetings were held on 'Attitudes to Mental Illness', and a film festival was organised where films such as *One Flew over the Cuckoo's Nest* were shown and discussed.

An important focus for much of this work has been the Community Planning Group (CPG) comprising local residents and users, supported by the community mental health worker. The planning group was established prior to the appointment of staff in order to ensure that the community had a voice in the development of the project. Its main aim is to act as a forum for local people and to reflect their needs and opinions. In practice it has also provided a way in which local residents can get together and become involved with Powell Street.

The CPG is formally organised with a chair, secretary, treasurer and a number of representatives who attend other meetings, such as meetings of the Community Health Council and meetings of the team and the Management Group. The CPG meets in a formal way every month and on average about 15 people attend. A smaller number of people attend the less formal weekly meetings when current business is discussed and an opportunity is provided for an exchange of information about activities.

Members of the CPG meet socially and have also organised social events for the wider community. These have included a barn dance and a 'beer and hot-pot supper'. In the future the CPG sees itself as having a major role to play in publicity, and in promoting mental health. The CPG has organised a regular coffee morning at the local community association. This provides a way of getting more people involved with Powell Street, and also provides a chance for CPG members to meet in a more informal atmosphere.

The CPG has access to money for training, which has provided opportunities for people to develop their skills and to visit other mental health developments. For example, members have attended courses at the local Community Education Centre and University, as well as national conferences organised by MIND and Community Health Action. The CPG has also been able to organise its own training programme. Many CPG members have found employment or have become involved with other local voluntary groups. The CPG are an important third party in the partnership with Health and Social Services. They have received many invitations to speak at conferences and requests to visit are received from other parts of the country. This suggests much interest in this model of community involvement.

Synthesis

'Powell Street' emerged in the wake of new definitions of mental health care and emerging government policies on care in the community. It is an attempt to synthesise elements emanating from new thinking and emerging policy and provides some insights into the rationale of this form of approach. It is worth reflecting on other models that are currently more prevalent within mental health and psychiatric services to illuminate the difference.

Most readers will be aware of the essential differences between local mental health services and more centralised services, which form the mainstream of provision. Table 3 highlights these. The contrast with existing services suggests that although it is in its early days the service that is emerging at Powell Street is different, not only in terms of its location but also its focus.

Community mental health services are now developing rapidly throughout the country. Although there is much diversity apparent in the philosophy and operation of these new services (Sayce, 1987) there are a number of common features and preoccupations. These include being locally based, an emphasis on community and consumer involvement, and the use of multiagency teams.

Table 3 Comparison between Powell Street and other health services for people with mental health problems

Dimension	Existing health services	Powell Street
Base	Based in hospitals (district general and psychiatric), health centres or day centres	Based in a residential street
Workers	Health or Social Services. May be working in 'teams' but unlikely to share accommodation or have common goals	Health and Social Services personnel organised in a team with joint management, sharing same site and having common aims and operational policy
Model	Primarily medical. Emphasis on individual pathology often reactive	Primarily sociological. Emphasis on social networks and integration. Reactive and proactive with emphasis on education
Target population	People with identifiable mental illness or mental health problems	People living in the defined geographic area
Referral	Usually via GP	Open—self-referrals encouraged
Activities	Residential day-time occupation. Individual support services often segregated	Non-residential groupwork—social networks Personal support. Community involvement. Emphasis on using existing resources and providing an integrated service
Consumer involvement	Few examples—the exception rather than the rule	Consumer involvement in management, service reviews and evaluation

Drawing briefly on the experience of Powell Street we wish to highlight these three themes.

Being locally based

One reason for decentralising services is to make them more accessible. 'Accessibility' is a concept that refers to more than just the physical location of a service. Other features of Powell Street — the informality, the open referral system, and the community profile — are designed to improve the accessibility of the service to local people in other ways. It has been suggested that sectorisation does not significantly alter the pattern of psychiatric services, but does allow a team to get to grips with the specific problems of a catchment area. From our experience being based locally does offer opportunities for a different type of service. These opportunities need to be grasped firmly if innovative practice is to be developed.

There has been a good opportunity to involve local people in the service. Mental health services historically have been set apart from the local community, and the consumers have been segregated. The presence of a locally based mental health project helps make mental health issues more visible. It increases the opportunity for people to get to know about what goes on in a mental health service and the people using the service are not so hidden from the local community.

Familiarity and developing relationships are potentially the most powerful ways of changing attitudes towards people who are seen as different. Working in the context in which people live means that workers are brought face to face with issues such as unemployment, poor housing and inadequate resources generally. This helps workers to see people in their family and social context, and strengthens a psychosocial view of mental health problems.

The fears, prejudices and labelling that form part of society's response to mental health problems must be weighed against these opportunities. Therefore, it was no surprise for us to realise that there is still stigma attached to Powell Street, and some people choose not to use such a local service, opting instead for the more distant hospital services. However, it is likely that this will change, albeit slowly, as local people build up their experience of our service, both as consumers and as local residents.

Community and consumer involvement

The experience of some people who become entangled with psychiatric services has been that even the most basic decisions are made on their behalf (for example, where to live, what time to get up and what to eat). Caught in a vicious circle, people not allowed to take control of their own destiny stand accused of not being capable of making decisions; this loss of autonomy is a characteristic feature of institutional life. The principles upon which Powell Street is based state that all people have the same rights regardless of disability (Brost et al., 1982) and the right of self-determination is seen as fundamental. The implication of this is that the service must be accountable to those people who use it. Powell Street has attempted to involve consumers in a sympathetic way in its operation (team meetings, management service review, training and evaluation), to promote people's self-determination in order to develop a service that is responsive.

However, therein lies a problem of definition; typically consumers are seen as those people who receive support on an individual basis. An emphasis on prevention means that community mental health services offer the possibility of redefinition, with the general public being viewed as potential or actual users of the service. Prevention of mental ill-health is a complicated idea and most authors now distinguish three types of prevention: primary, secondary and tertiary. Primary prevention is the least precisely defined term, but it is usually taken to mean the reduction in the occurrence of new cases of people with mental health problems and the development of competence as protection against mental ill-health (Koch, 1986). Secondary prevention refers to the earlier identification and intervention with people whose problems have not become long-standing. Tertiary prevention aims to reduce the residual effects of long-term mental health problems and is more usually the domain of traditional mental health services. Powell Street aims to work on all three levels, which means that both people with well-established mental health problems and members of the community at large are invited to participate, and are not actively differentiated as consumers and non-consumers. This should be read in the context of research carried out by Goldberg and Huxley (1980), which suggested that the psychiatric morbidity detected by specialist services, and even at the primary care level, was significantly less than that present in the community at large. We are aware from information from local people that some people do not seek help because of the process of labelling that this entails — it is therefore important that people are able to participate in the service without this happening.

The participation of the community in the service also helps with integration. Building up local people's experience of people with mental health problems was seen as a prerequisite for more tolerant communities by those planning Powell Street. The CPG is a start, although it is clear that in all our activities there have to be some safeguards against the social processes of marginalisation that can occur.

Multiagency Working

It now seems to be generally accepted in the field of mental health that multiagency teams represent the way forward.

Powell Street was established as a jointly funded, jointly managed service, shared between Health and Social Services. We have always believed broad representation to be important since potentially it offers a wide range of information, opinion, ideas and choice for the consumer. However, two major issues arise which will need further debate.

These are, firstly, the relevance in a setting such as described above, of the skills of the traditional multiagency team, and the accessibility of skilled workers to local people.

Secondly, in a multiagency team, there are at least two employing organisations to be considered, each with their own professional and bureaucratic rules. The position of a team's staff within their own hierarchy is usually relatively powerless. Fieldworkers in both Health and Social Services Departments usually have little direct access to decision-making processes and are in a position of dual accountability to their clients and to their employers. Organisational interests may not coincide with those of the individual.

This conflict of interests may become particularly problematic where a service claims to 'give power to the people' but does not in reality invest much of that power in the workers, who may be the only people in a position to implement power sharing.

These are issues that require further consideration if services are to be truly local, responsive and participative.

Concluding Comments

It has been argued that new services are long overdue. Powell Street is an attempt to provide a new service that is planned around people's lives in the community. As it has developed it has aimed to be responsive and accountable to the people who use the service and to the wider community. This model of service development needs to be viewed as a partial response to a political policy geared towards the resettlement of people from the long-stay hospitals where inadequate attention may be paid to their lives in the community.

References

Brost, M., and Johnson, T. (1982). *Getting to Know You: One Approach to Service Assessment and Planning for Individuals with Disabilities.* Wisconsin.

Finch, J., and Groves, D. (1983) *A Labour of Love. Women, Work and Care.* Routledge and Kegan Paul, London.

Goldberg, D.T., and Huxley, T.J. (1980) *Mental Illness in the Community: The Pathway to Psychiatric Care.* Tavistock, London.

Gray, J. (1985) 'Planning for Individuals', in McAusland, T. (ed.) *Planning and Monitoring Community Mental Health Centres.* King's Fund Centre, London.

Hagan, T. (1987) Personal communication.

Koch, H. (1986) 'Anxiety and Depression. A Community Mental Health Perspective', In Koch, H. (ed.) *Community Clinical Psychology.* Croom Helm, London.

Malin, N. (1987) 'Community Care: Principles, Policies and Practice', in Malin, N. (ed.) *Re-assessing Community Care.* Croom Helm, London.

MIND (1986) Report of an Evaluative Visit to 2 Powell Street, Community Mental Health Service, Clayton. Unpublished.

Openshaw Outreach Mental Health Project (1984) North Manchester Health Authority. Unpublished.

Sayce, L. (ed.) (1987) *Community Mental Health Centres. Report of the annual conference 1987.* National Unit for Psychiatric Research and Development, in collaboration with Good Practices in Mental Health.

Wolfensberger, W. (1972) *The Principle of Normalisation in Human Services.* NIMR. Toronto.

Wolfensberger, W., and Glenn, L. (1975) PASS 3 – *Program Analysis of Service Systems,* 3rd Edition. NIMR. Toronto.

Changing Ideas in Health Care
Edited by D. Seedhouse and A. Cribb
© 1989 John Wiley & Sons Ltd

Chapter Nine
North Manchester: Women's Health at Risk

SALLY CAWLEY, ANGELA MARTIN, ANN INMAN and PAM MUTTRAM
Women's Health Team
Newton Heath
Manchester
UK

Introduction

North Manchester's Women's Health Team is the first permanently funded specialist NHS service of its kind in the country providing a radical approach to preventive health care for women. It is a service that aims to incorporate the philosophies from the women's health movement into day-to-day practice in order to respond to the needs and demands of women in North Manchester.

The Women's Health Team works within a feminist philosophy that acknowledges a woman's right to a more holistic consideration of her health. The team rejects the 'victim blaming' approach and seeks to give control back to the woman, and the confidence to express her health needs as an equal with others.

Since its inception in 1985 the Women's Health Team has been regarded by many as a 'definitive' model of 'Well Women' provision. The team is constantly approached by voluntary and statutory agencies throughout Britain to outline guidelines for establishing similar NHS-based services. The working reality shows that the model is not perfect. There are many lessons to be derived from the frustrating experience of trying to work in an innovative way inside the massive hierarchical bureaucracy of the NHS.

Progress in North Manchester

The impact of the women's health movement in this country and the concomitant rise of nationwide women's health courses, self-help/support groups and Well Women Clinics has been documented elsewhere (Orr, 1987). The North Manchester experience has to be seen in this overall context. A combination of powerful personalities, community interest and support, some receptive health authority members, Community Health Council pressure and a climate of growing political awareness of women's health issues led in 1983 to the creation of the Women's Health Project.

The Women's Health Project

In North Manchester the specialist in community medicine and the District Medical Officer were committed to providing community health care for sections of the community whose health was most at risk in an inner city area. Both women had been involved in establishing Well Women Clinics in the south of the city and wished to see a more broad-based approach implemented in the North district. In order to assess the viability of a new service, a research project was funded for one year by the Manpower Services Commission. Amongst its recommendations was the establishment of the present Women's Health Team.

The project set out to evaluate a Mobile Well Women Industrial Screening Service and considered proposals for a similar 'in-house' NHS screening system. It assessed the health needs of women in the district and consulted them and the health workers about service proposals. The workers were involved in research into the rate of take-up of cervical screening, in collaboration with the University of Manchester. They also played a public relations and developmental role that involved liaison with groups and agencies in the area, acknowledging existing health initiatives as well as identifying gaps in the service provided to the community. The overall aim was to listen to the needs that the community identified, rather than to impose a service based on theory or good intention.

Three part-time research workers were employed at the outset. Staffing was increased six months later when two workers with a community development role joined the team. Unfortunately, the workers encountered problems of isolation due to the location of the team in the large district hospital. The project was poorly funded and had little status in relation to mainstream services. The nature of the project, and the types of body to which it was accountable, meant that workers felt it continually necessary to produce reports designed to break down resistance to the acceptance of women's health as a central issue.

The project's major achievements included: the establishment of a Well Women Resource Bank; the forging of community links and networks with individual women and groups — both locally and nationally; the move towards a more 'woman centred' approach to women's health care — a challenge to the medical model of provision; the writing of a number of reports; proposals (Proposals for the Promotion of Preventive Health Services for Women in the North District — June 1984, Unpublished) that recommended, after extensive community and professional consultation, the establishment of a central Well Women Resource Centre, associated Well Women Centres and a specialist team of workers to carry out preventive health care in North Manchester.

The project finished in September 1984 and negotiations began in order to implement the recommendations and discuss funding options. An application for Urban Aid money from central government was successful and the health authority agreed to contribute the other two-thirds of a total annual budget of approximately £32,000.

The Urban Aid money was granted until April 1987, at which point the health authority was committed to meeting the continuation costs, thus ensuring that the team and centre once set up would become a recognised mainstream community unit service. Once the decision to fund the service had been made low cost premises were designated and the building refurbished to house the resource centre.

The Formation of a Team

In May 1985 the workers' posts were advertised alongside three senior health promotion posts as North Manchester's new Health Promotion Unit was created. The decision was made to link the workers to Health Promotion as the proposed style of fieldworking appeared to have more relevance to a unit committed to a community development approach. It seemed that a co-ordinated approach to preventive primary health care was set to make significant changes in the district's health profile.

In July 1985 three part-time health promotion officers (scale 4) and a part-time clerical/administration worker were employed to form a specialist team within the community unit to act as a focus for the development of responsive health services for women. The team's brief was to establish a resource and information centre, produce and disseminate health resources, to liaise with NHS staff and other statutory and voluntary agencies, and to support women's initiatives in the community and in the developing satellite Well Women Clinics throughout the district.

Until January 1987 the team was managed by and professionally accountable to the Health Promotion Unit. It was intended that this arrangement would enable the team to be part of mainstream health promotion discussions. In turn this would allow the fieldworkers to feed the demands of the women they worked with back into the mainstream system. However, the management structure for the team had been omitted from the original proposals and this led to a lack of clarity over role and accountability: this was a constant source of frustration for the workers.

It is clear to the team that unless community health initiatives have access to a structure that can actually implement identified community needs, projects can become marginalised and can lose credibility. One of the main advantages of community health initiatives being within the NHS is that they should have more power to effect change in generic services. Nothing can be achieved if the system closes its doors to new and challenging ideas.

The Women's Health Team pressed at an early stage for a more senior forum of NHS management to be set up to consider the overall policy for women's health services in the district. The District Planning Group for Women's Health Services now exists under the chair of the District Medical Officer. A wide range of NHS professionals come together each month to develop strategies of primary health care for North Manchester women. This planning group should ensure that existing structures are challenged and that new initiatives operate within a supportive management framework.

The team is currently managed by the Area II primary care manager with formalised supervision from the Senior Health Promotion Officer for education. This has been found to be a more serviceable arrangement. Two women psychologists from the district hold monthly review sessions for the workers concerning issues that arise during the weekly drop-in sessions at the centre. The reviews provide a valuable forum for the workers to evaluate critically their skills and to support each other around particularly difficult issues that may arise during the regular drop-in sessions.

Developing a Team Approach

The work of the team draws on resource, information, community development, youth work and publicity skills, as well as the less formalised listening and communication skills of the workers. It has always been a priority to budget for training in order to enable the workers to develop these skills and expand into new areas. Workers have attended and led workshops at national and regional conferences. They have also invited trainers and experienced women to lead sessions at the centre that are attended by the workers themselves and by other NHS community staff.

Work practice and the general direction of the team has developed in accordance with the skills and interests of the workers. Since the workers come from a variety of work backgrounds, and have had different personal experiences, a broad-based service has been created. An early part of the workers' induction involved a trip to London to visit other projects with a similar brief, as well as visits to more locally based groups working with women. These national and local contacts formed the basis of a comprehensive women's health network.

New services often neglect the need to establish an identity, address the workers' needs and anxieties, and to plan initial development strategies because of pressure to be seen to be achieving something. One of the most important aspects of the Women's Health Team's early work was to break down suspicion amongst the statutory services, and to validate community development methods of working in women's health. This was a high priority, and had to be done before any visible progress could be made.

The time spent learning to work creatively and collectively as a team has been a major strength of the workers, particularly in more recent times when funding has been threatened.

The first five months were a period of liaison and networking whilst the workers set up the centre and publicised their plans and existence to women, agencies and groups in the district and nationally. It was also the time to get to know each other, to learn to work together collectively and to define the aims and objectives that would become the foundation from which the daily work could be evaluated, and a philosophy of women's health developed.

The aims and objectives are constantly reviewed so that flexibility and change in work practice are encouraged. This process is preferred to conventional attempts to meet quantitative targets, which the team regards as restrictive. The quality of the service is considered to be more important than its conformity to rigid criteria of success or failure.

It could be argued that community health projects should create a new and more appropriate language of evaluation, one that reflects the nature of community participation in health care. At an early stage the team approached a group of feminist women researchers in Manchester to act as consultants for this new style of evaluation. The consultants worked alongside the team at development meetings to clarify the following aims and objectives that the team had identified. Needless to say not all of these have been fully addressed to date.

1. To create a safe 'women only' space, where women have time to talk and share experiences.
2. To provide a welcoming and accessible service to all women.
3. To provide free childcare at all services used by women.
4. To address issues of race, culture and racism, disability and access, sexuality, discrimination and negative attitudes towards younger and older women in all areas of the team's work.
5. To provide women with good clear health information.
6. To encourage and promote liaison and co-operation with other agencies to ensure a co-ordinated approach to preventive health services for women.
7. To provide a focus for women's health initiatives in North Manchester and to develop channels to feed identified needs back to improve provision in the health service and other relevant agencies.
8. To establish the Women's Health Team as an integral part of mainstream service provision by securing a realistic budget that allows for consolidation and further growth.

These aims have changed over time and will change again as the service adapts to reflect the information it gains from women in the community.

The Centre

In order that the centre could fulfil its aims to be accessible to all women, the team had to ensure that women with babies and young chldren were not prevented from coming to the drop-in sessions. When the centre first opened in January 1986 a creche worker was employed to cover the drop-in sessions, all events, and daytime discussion groups. The creche worker is part of the team and has a developmental role reviewing resources, giving talks at local nurseries and being involved in all the team's events. Free childcare at all NHS facilities should be the norm and it has always been a priority in Well Women provision. As from 1988, the community unit will be ensuring free creche provision in more of its clinics, in a mental health day care centre, in other community health projects, and in all Well Women services.

The service operates outside the traditional model of medical health care and as such needed a base that was informal and would not be too closely associated with more clinical or statutory provision. An ideal location would probably have been a shop front in a local shopping area or in a house in one of the large estates in North Manchester. However, the resource centre is based in a small house attached to the Baby Clinic in Pilling Street, Newton Heath, away from the main road. The building was designated by the health authority as the most financially viable option and was chosen on these grounds rather than through consultation with a local community. Consequently it is in a fairly isolated situation and is not in an area normally identified with community activity. It could be argued that since the health team is to serve the district the neighbourhood aspect was of lesser importance, and indeed statistics show that hundreds of women and professionals have used the centre since it opened in January 1986. However, the team has always felt that the service is too small to respond adequately to district needs, and yet does not have sufficient roots in a local community to be a neighbourhood only service.

The centre itself has a warm relaxed feel to it. The downstairs room is furnished as a living room with comfortable chairs and the small kitchen provides extra space when the centre is busy. Women who have used it say it feels very 'homely'.

The centre has several functions. It provides office space for the workers, a meeting room for women's groups, a phone line for women who cannot come to the centre or who prefer to make contact by phone, and has a resource and information bank that is probably the most extensive outside London. It also provides space for a regular drop-in session and women's support group.

The resources are available to any women who live and work in North Manchester. To serve the ever-increasing demand the centre offers a wide range of resources; free leaflets and factsheets written from women's experiences, leaflets from the team, the excellent material developed by the Women's Health Information Centre in London and Adelaide (Australia) Women's Health Group, and a selection of women's health books, video- and audio-tapes, which are available for loan.

Information on the menopause is the most frequently requested item. Both individual women and groups of women have asked the team for information and contacts to lead discussion sessions. In response to this demand the Women's Health Team asked the two women psychologists to work with them to set up menopause support groups. Unfortunately, these groups did not get off the ground, mainly because in the two neighbourhoods selected there was no access to other community-based workers who might have publicised the groups existence and encouraged women to become involved.

Other issues that women identify are stress and depression, lack of information about cervical screening, period problems and PMT, cancer, domestic stress and violence, skin disorders, and inappropriate or insensitive responses from GPs, hospital or other statutory services.

Most of the requests come from women who live or work in the district. However, the team also receives a high proportion of calls from outside the health authority boundaries, often as a result of publicity on local radio or in the *Manchester Evening News*. Where possible women are referred to a group or a Well Women Clinic in their area, but the workers will often spend time listening to the woman on the telephone if she does not have anywhere else to take her problem.

The centre is increasingly being utilised by other community health staff who want to use more appropriate resources with the women they come into contact with. A considerable amount of worker time is spent with students and other visitors to the centre, explaining its function and showing them how best to utilise the resources.

One of the most important functions of the centre is to act as a referral point both to and from other agencies, support groups and NHS services. Good relationships have been developed with other North Manchester clinics, women nurses in the Community Psychiatric Nursing Team, women psychologists, Community Education, and Community Development, as well as with the numerous groups in the voluntary sector throughout Greater Manchester.

Production and dissemination of written information is one of the most time-consuming aspects of the work, and the administration tasks required to maintain and develop the centre were underestimated in the original budget. If a community health project of this kind is to have a secure base from which to expand it needs an adequate budget for resources and staffing, which must include sufficient clerical and administrative support.

A Continuing Struggle

Statutory sector projects are often assumed to be free from funding difficulties common to voluntary sector groups. The Women's Health Team fought for two years to gain access to monies to secure a budget that would increase the workers' hours to full-time, and more recently has been under constant pressure to prove its right to exist within a National Health Service that seems increasingly hostile to preventive health care as government cuts decimate already run-down services.

As from April 1987, the team has been reduced from four to three workers. Even though the remaining health promotion officers have shared their colleague's 20 hours between them the loss of a worker has caused added strain and more work for individuals in the team. It has also reduced dynamism. A team of four was able to generate far more in the way of political challenge and ideas than three workers have been able to do. This has led to frustration as many ideas now are not realised due to lack of woman power.

The planning and running of special events that aim to promote women's health as something to be enjoyed and also to raise awareness of the impact of women's social, political and emotional environment on their well-being, has been directly affected by the insufficient funding. The themes that have been possible have included pregnancy and motherhood, (for which Manchester's Contact Theatre's production 'The Baby Show' was hired) and healthy eating and additives (during this day workers prepared additive-free health foods, and recipes were typed out and made available to women). Sexual harassment was tackled by the Sheffield-based theatre company, the Chuffinelles, and the issue of women and violence was further reinforced by a Health Day at a local neighbourhood centre, which made domestic violence and abuse of power the main theme. Earlier in the year the team arranged for NE1 Theatre from Newcastle to perform a play about incest and sexual abuse in two venues. The team ensured that support systems were available for women of any age who needed to talk after the Theatre-in-Education piece had brought back memories of abuse for them.

Everyone involved sees these events as vital catalysts for health awareness, and the response from women has been very encouraging. However, the money to stage these popular events has generally come from other agencies: Community Development and the Equal Opportunities Units of Manchester City Council were the major contributors. The team's 1987/8 budget now allows for a special events pool of money and will enable continuation of this work.

Using the Centre

Once a week, on a Tuesday afternoon, the centre is open for women to drop in to chat with the workers and other users about health concerns. This informal session takes place in the downstairs 'living-room' where written resources are available for women to look through. The workers are able to spend time with all the women present. Rooms are available upstairs for women who prefer to talk with a worker in private.

An average of between six and eight women use these sessions each week. The small living-room and kitchen have been packed with as many as 20 women on a particularly busy day. At these sessions the regular users play an important role making sure that those who have come for the first time feel welcome and at ease.

The weekly afternoon session runs for three hours, so women do not feel pressurised to rush their conversation and workers have time to listen. At the end of each session the workers hold a 'debriefing' session, for time together to wind down and for support. During the session the workers are around to listen to women and to help them find the most appropriate resource, in the form of information or referral. For many women having the time to talk about themselves within a safe, confidential, non-judgemental setting can be the most important aspect. The most frequent feedback the team receives is 'It's the first time anyone has ever really listened' and 'Until I talked to other women I thought I was the only one who felt like this'.

Physical and emotional isolation are two powerful and insidious determinants of women's ill-health. By helping women to feel more confident about articulating their needs and making choices about their health, the team tries to enable them to regain control of situations and relationships in which they often feel powerless.

Most of the women who use the centre come alone. Others bring a friend or relative, and the drop-ins often have groups of women arriving by minibus from community centres throughout the district. It takes a lot of courage to ask for help and many of the women who use the centre are doing so as a last resort because other systems of care have failed them in some way.

> Whilst following my career I frequently experienced symptoms which caused me great distress, I decided to seek help from my GP. I had panic attacks which were quite frightening and after prescribing many drugs but no verbal help I realised I was not improving, the doctor said it was an anxiety state and finally suggested that I see a Psychiatrist. After much treatment with Group Therapy and Psychologists I did improve but was looking for friendly help, this I found at the Well Women's Centre, seeing it advertised I decided to give it a try although with little faith. The welcome I found from a small group was unbelievable and restored much of my confidence. I have found friendship and help which I continue to get. My panic attacks are less frequent and with the help of a counsellor I have reduced my drug intake to a minimum which has been quite difficult. I now feel that I'm on the road to recovery.
>
> (S. Gregory, Newton Heath)

Many of the women who come to the Pilling Street centre come because they feel they have reached a point of health crisis. Being able to share this experience, to be listened to with empathy and respect, and to be able to consider a range of choices can prove a watershed in giving the women a chance to take back some control. The majority only come once or twice but for others the centre has come to represent a 'safe' place where they can come each week to relax and chat to the workers and other women.

Friendships have been made at the centre, and women have been encouraged to be involved in producing their own resources based on their personal experience. For example, a 'panic attack' leaflet is currently being printed. It will be a valuable resource, and there is a further benefit in that the women who wrote it found that putting their experiences on paper has helped their anxieties.

However the 'safety-net' function of the centre has changed the role of the workers, who have become much more involved with counselling rather than with the group work skills required to facilitate more general preventive work. This has meant considerable extra stress for the workers since the centre's drop-ins aim to provide an informal listening, help and information service and not formalised counselling. Where appropriate, women are referred to specialist counselling agencies. The team works very closely with the women psychologists and Community Psychiatric Nurses (CPNs), the latter are now taking self-referrals from women who have visited the centre and want tranquilliser withdrawal programmes.

Issues that have arisen out of the contact of workers with women have greatly influenced the development of the team's concept of service provision and the role of the centre. One of the main needs articulated was for a regular weekly group where the same women could get together for support.

In Janury 1987 the Women's Health Team publicised and started the Wednesday Group which meets weekly for two hours in the afternoon. Run jointly by a member of the Women's Health Team and a counsellor from North Manchester College, it functions as a group for women who need support and help through a variety of problems. After a slow start the sessions began to flourish. A core group of ten regular members, found it a helpful forum for discussion, enabling them to gain more self-confidence.

'If you had seen me when I first came to the group — you just wouldn't have believed it was the same person.'

'It [the group] gives me a reason for getting up and dressed — it really is a great help to me.'

'I wouldn't keep coming if I didn't think it was doing me some good'.

It would appear that the Wednesday Group has acted as a springboard for some of the women who have moved on to more challenging ventures. One woman has joined an information technology course whilst another has been involved in the training for volunteer workers in the Well Women Centre in Cheetham.

Numbers in the group vary as women find other involvements and new members join. The programme includes trips out (some of the women in the group are agoraphobic and have found the outings great confidence boosters). There are also relaxation afternoons as well as discussion sessions.

The Wednesday Group is a valuable example of group preventive mental health care work and the team would like to see more support groups of this kind in the district.

The development of each of the team's ventures has depended on good publicity about the aims and availability of the service. Women have contacted the team as a result of both the extensive formal publicity and the passing of information by word-of-mouth — 'I got talking to a woman on the bus and told her I was worried about this lump. She said she'd been to the Well Women's and she felt much better.'

Good, clearly written publicity has been a priority from the start. Fortunately, layout and design skills were available in the team and the women's health service leaflets with their distinctive 'cartoon women' are instantly recognisable. The leaflets encourage women and local workers to use the whole range of services on offer.

Despite constantly reviewing this vital work (work that is not common to other NHS services — many of which seem determined to surround themselves with such mystery that they become inaccessible), having good local media coverage, and undertaking door-to-door leafleting, the team are still not reaching enough women. Black women, older women, women with disabilities and young women have traditionally been ignored and ill-served by the NHS and an early priority was to consider issues raised for these women in all aspects of the team's work.

Work with Girls and Young Women

Open, accessible health information, resources, advice and services for young women are few and far between. Young women's needs and concerns are diverse.

Many young women have little knowledge of the way their bodies work, about menstruation or any of the other physical and emotional changes that are part of young womanhood. There is very little good information about sex, sexuality and contraception. So many young women find it difficult to put their own needs first in relationships. There is also a growing number of teenage 'unplanned' pregnancies — and a lack of services and support for either continuing or terminating them; and there is fear of AIDS and other sexually transmitted diseases. In a lot of cases young women have nowhere and no-one to turn to for non-judgemental support when suffering the pressures and stresses that these issues raise, or to talk through the many other aspects of living that affect their health and well-being.

The Women's Health Team has always placed particular emphasis on both providing and supporting the growth of more points of access where young women *can* talk, get support and good clear information. A wide range of resources has been built up (videos, leaflets, books and games) for use in raising awareness of girls and young women to health and health-related issues. The day-to-day work has taken a variety of approaches to respond to the diverse needs of girls and young women and (where appropriate) to the women who are working with them. The team ran a highly successful 'Girls Health Stall' at Manchester Girls' Day to celebrate International Women's Week in March 1987. This provided an opportunity to talk to young women about specific health issues and about where they could find more general resources and services. Such events also provide an opportunity to make contact with youth workers and teachers who may want to start or develop their own health work. The team has run sessions for established groups of young women, in their youth clubs and schools, and also at the centre. Training sessions with youth workers have sometimes been general — for example an 'open' session to screen and discuss a video on menstruation recently made by some young women in Liverpool — but more often they are specific requests from individual workers or teams from different centres. Growing numbers of young women are coming to the open sessions at the centre and raising as wide a range of issues as any other age group.

The team attaches great importance to raising the profile of girls' and young women's concerns within the women's and community health fields; endeavouring to do this regionally and nationally as well as in North Manchester. We have also run workshops at Well Women and community health conferences.

At a time of cuts in the education sector and with the introduction of Mr Baker's Education Act, the innovative work that is being developed both within the team and by youth workers and teachers in the area is in danger of being pushed off the agenda. The team are anxious to help maintain and support such work whenever and wherever possible — but NHS resources are similarly limited.

It is perhaps surprising to outsiders that a city the size of Manchester has no Brook Advisory Service or other specialist young people's health provision. Now that the Women's Health Team is established and has developed valuable networks amongst young women and workers, this must be the next stage in making better provision for young women's needs. Liaison between the health authority, the local education authority and the voluntary sector is essential if services are to be open, accessible and genuinely responsive. There is no doubt at all that the needs, the ideas and the enthusiasm abound — but the availability of essential resources is, sadly, way behind.

Older Women, Disability and Carers

Lack of resources is a recurrent theme in the life of any community health project and inevitably dictates the pace at which services can develop — prioritising certain areas of work has meant that others must suffer and the team are keenly aware that they have never had the 'woman-hours' adequately to address the needs of older women and women with disabilities.

The team has spent a lot of time pushing for adequate access to the community clinics it has been involved in. This has resulted in the completion of a ramp but has not profoundly changed attitudes to the point at which it is accepted that making buildings physically accessible to everyone is only a first step.

It is the voluntary sector that is making the more radical steps in campaigning for the needs of women caring for elderly and dependent relatives. The team's role was to be part of a process of bringing other workers together to begin a dialogue of collaboration and co-operation.

Two carers' support groups have subsequently been set up offering emotional and practical support for carers in two areas of North Manchester. It feels a very piecemeal approach to major issues but it is a very important area of work since the team's community development, fieldwork and work with individual women can be nothing more than 'patching the cracks' if work aimed at raising awareness within the system is not effective.

An 'A–Z' for Carers was produced by a multidisciplinary group of workers and women involved with carers in conjunction with a very successful Carers Fair, which focused on exploring and publicising issues for carers in North Manchester. The 'A–Z' was co-ordinated by the Association of Carers and the Women's Health Team, and funded by the Community Health Council.

Work with Asian Women/Community Development Work

A high percentage of the population in the Cheetham Hill area of North Manchester are non-white. There are many Asian families and people of other ethnic origins whose health needs are not being met by the existing health and statutory services.

Part of the team's brief was to develop women's health services in this area. The women who had been actively campaigning for several years for a Well Women Centre soon made their demands known. The women wanted a centre that would be run by local women for local women outside the medical model of provision, but with the services of a woman doctor.

The team approached non-white women workers and activists involved in the area to clarify whether the proposed provision would meet their needs and to begin discussion about the health needs of the Asian community.

During the meetings that followed a decision was made to hold a Health Day for women and that this should be done in conjunction with the women already involved in the Well Women campaign and other workers in the area who had shown an interest in women's health care provision.

The day was organised in the context of overall discussion about improving services for women in Cheetham and with the stated aim of making the needs of Asian women a priority. It was imperative that the day linked women to existing services in the community as well as opening up new community health possibilities for all women.

Planning meetings were held for nine months with local women and involved workers. All publicity and some leaflets were in Urdu and English, and Asian women made themselves available on the day to translate and interpret where necessary. The planning group were keenly aware of the inadequacies of provision of health information both culturally and linguistically on the day and has since pushed for better district resources in languages other than English.

Over 100 women came to the Health Day where the emphasis was on information and practical preventive health care. Stalls included: sickle cell, herbal teas, nutrition and breast feeding. A questionnaire in Urdu and English was used to get an idea of what issues women would wish to pursue after the day. Women who completed the form indicated a wide range of topics. As a result the local further education college and TUBE were approached for funding and two health courses were set up: one for Asian women during the day-time (run by an Asian woman counsellor and a white women's health tutor) and an evening course for any woman run by another white women's health tutor.

Both the courses that originated from the day were successful, particularly the Asian women's course. This course allowed many of the women to articulate their feelings that their ill health is caused by institutionalised racism and inadequate service provision. Mental ill-health, depression and stress were the main themes running through both courses.

The Asian women were clear that they wanted to continue with the sessions, and another two courses (both day-time) began a few months later. This time the Asian women's course was co-ordinated by two women from within the community. The counsellor from the previous course took on a more prominent role.

All ages of women came to share experiences and the group now has its own status and is approaching the college and other agencies for further funding. The group has also been involved with the team in campaigning for an Asian women's health worker. The health authority have responded by submitting an Urban Programme Bid but the women are clear that they also want to explore other alternatives. A large group of interested workers and other women are currently meeting to consider options for an Asian women's health worker (with broad-based management and support) who would have an outreach and development role providing a much-needed voice for the women's demands.

The role of the Women's Health Team worker with the Asian Women's Health Group has been to open up access to funding and resources, to offer encouragement and support for initiatives and to ensure that the issues raised were fed back to the health authority through the District Planning Group for Women's Health Services and also to local health services managers. The women in Cheetham, active in discussion, are clear that local health services must be improved and that the Well Women provision is a complement and not an alternative.

Well Women Centres And Clinics

In April 1987 the Cheetham Well Women Centre opened after a ten-week training programme for the volunteer workers, who were drawn from the original planning group. The centre has had a lot of problems with premises and is now located on the city council's community development double decker bus. This provides a highly visual and unusual venue attracting many passing women. However, more permanent premises are urgently needed so that women have a centre they feel they can be more involved in.

A second group of women is currently undergoing training, which is being co-ordinated by the Women's Health Team but is run and jointly devised by the volunteer workers from the first programme. As new women become involved on the bus they are encouraged to participate in training if they show an interest. The main focus of the training is challenging prejudice and assumptions, and equipping the women with information-giving and listening skills whilst building their confidence and increasing their existing skills.

The future of the service looks promising. It provides a model for community initiated Well Women Centres and demonstrates how a district-wide service such as the Women's Health Team can respond to women's demands on a neighbourhood basis through local participation, negotiation and discussion.

In 1986 the team worked closely with Beswick Women's Health Group running courses and a Health Day. The following year workers involved with the group applied for funding for a women's health worker for the Beswick area.

The Women's Health Clinic in Beswick was the first in the district. Community health visitors and the Clinical Medical Officer (CMO) were not satisfied with merely changing the name of the cytology sessions to a Well Women session but wanted to create a more responsive service for women. The Women's Health Team has worked with the Beswick staff mainly in a support and resourcing capacity. To date the team has co-run two training courses for community health nurses in women's health issues, largely as a response to pressure from Beswick HVs but also as an attempt to open up this way of working to as many generic staff as possible.

The Beswick clinic has been offering the clinical role that the Women's Health Team workers, who are not medically trained, could not. During the planning phase for the team's structure it was felt that a non-clinical team would provide an alternative, more open, non-threatening environment for women. Yet it soon became apparent that there was a need for clinical services for the team to refer to so that women had a chance to explore fully their physical as well as mental health needs. Beswick had always taken referrals from, and referred women to the team, but huge demand had begun to put too much pressure on the Beswick workers. Also the clinic was two or more bus rides away for women from other neighbourhoods, so it was imperative to look at the possibility of setting up more Well Women Clinics.

In August 1986 a new CMO was appointed who had a particular interest and a lot of experience in women's health work. She commented:

> From the beginning I have found it made a big difference to my work to be able to inform women about the drop-in sessions at Pilling Street. Many women come to cytology and family planning sessions with problems around the menopause, pre-menstrual tension etc. Often while exploring the reasons for heavy periods or increases in hot flushes, for example, women will bring up problems that they are trying to cope with. In a busy clinic session I can only skim over the surface of these problems. For these women I often give them the information about the drop-in sessions and explain what they can expect, having full confidence that one of the workers will be able to spend more time allowing the woman to explore these issues, and helping her make the connections between her life situation and her health. In most cases I do not formally refer women, but leave it to them to make the contact as and when they need it.

Much of this work, which took place during regular family planning and cytology sessions, had clear implications for more formalised provision. Once the need was established, a new Women's Health Clinic started at the Community Clinic next door to the Women's Health Team base. Pilling Street health visitors expressed an interest in working with the CMO to establish a monthly session.

The session has proved to be extremely popular with women who have been encouraged to refer themselves by the team, and the numbers have been so high that most sessions have run long past the allocated two hours. Discussions took place at Women's Health Clinic workers' meetings (convened by the Women's Health Team) as to the viability of evening sessions but the heavy demands on health service staff has meant this much-needed service for both clinical and non-clinical sessions has not evolved.

Other CMOs have been encouraged to be involved in women's health issues and the team receives referrals from CMOs and a few GPs. In line with all Well Women services the CMOs cannot prescribe drugs and must refer the woman back to her own GP, but they can offer the time that GPs often cannot.

The CMO involved in the monthly Well Women session, in conjunction with Cheetham Well Women Centre, underwent the same training as the volunteers in an attempt at team building and to address issues of power and equal skill sharing. The CMO involved at Pilling Street Clinic has also been involved in co-training with the Women's Health Team worker in Cheetham and has done important networking with her colleagues and at district planning level. 'I have thoroughly enjoyed working with the Women's Health Team. Coming from a common philosophy, and being able to share our very different skills, has been very creative for me, and for the women we have worked with.'

The overall provision of women's health services within the district should be regarded as a complementary service to the work that goes on amongst other community health staff. The Women's Health Team hopes to support and publicise other workers' initiatives and to provide a focal point for resourcing and exchange of ideas.

It is also important that the development of clinics is seen in the context of the other work of the team as the clinics are generally only the visible manifestation of months of community development and liaison work. The one cannot exist without the other, and recognition of an often laborious way of working is vital if the work is not to be marginalised.

Conclusions

Women's health issues should be on everyone's agenda, from community nurses to policy-making managers. The team has often spoken of a feeling of being the 'conscience of local NHS provision' taking on and prioritising issues of race, gender and sexuality, and challenging the lack of any real commitment to change within the NHS. The main success of the team as part of the NHS must be judged by the degree to which the issues raised by women through the team have been responded to and reflected in more appropriate service provision.

The team feels that 'change from within' is possible since there are many health workers keen and committed to new ways of working, but, financial cutbacks have made the realisation of that commitment difficult.

Most community health projects seem to have taken a couple of years to establish themselves, after $2\frac{1}{2}$ years it feels that the Women's Health Team is now a recognised part of local NHS provision, gaining support from women and workers in the district, and is finally beginning to feel secure.

The project, at time of writing, has entered a phase of consolidation and whilst this will ultimately prove to be valuable it has occurred because of low staffing levels and not because on-going evaluation has shown the need to halt development at this point. The project was instigated with a 'phased development' structure — it is imperative that the structure is capable of growth even in later phases.

The crucial networking of the early months continues, particularly within the NHS, in an attempt to create a more receptive health environment for women. Alongside this, the more radical developmental and outreach work prevents the project becoming a token gesture: a sticking plaster to keep women from challenging the inequalities in the system — rather the team's work is often a catalyst to activity.

The demand for the service has been proven and evaluation that incorporates women's experiences and workers' skills and sets them in the context of NHS constraints, has allowed for flexibility and responsiveness in the service and has enabled workers to explore new ways of working. The project evaluates its work for an audience that includes local women users, the workers themselves, other community health projects, managers and the health authority. By focusing on process, and not on rigid quantitative determinants of success and failure, the project's achievements can be seen in a philosophical, political and economic context — one that reflects the lives of the women the project has worked with.

Under the present government there is little point in being naive about the future of the team or its ability to promote a preventive health care model that treats women's health as the norm. However, the potential of such a team is enormous and if it received sufficient financial support to explore the developments outlined then the team could play a part in making North Manchester a healthier place for women. Proposed areas of work for the future include:

1. The expansion of the team and the more effective implementation of the equal opportunity employment policy.
2. Securing an expanded resource budget. The Women's Health Team has the most comprehensive resource centre outside London — in order to maintain and refine the system money needs to be put into new resources.
3. Developing resources (an area that, so far, has been neglected) particularly jointly producing material like the 'Women and AIDS' leaflet, which was written in conjunction with the Health Promotion Unit.

   Producing resources that consider women's diversity — being sensitive to race and ethnic background; sensory, physical and mental disability; sexual orientation; domestic and economic situation; age; and literacy. This would include the provision of health information on cassette.

   Working with local non-white women's groups and the Health Promotion Unit to translate existing materials.

   Ensuring that literature produced is distributed through health centres, clinics and community centres.
4. Reviewing the team's training role so that the workers' skills are appropriately used, and ensuring that there is no confusion over training that should be carried out by others. The team is keen to work with generic community nurses and student nurses in the context of an environment that supports new work and furthers the commitment to expanding Women's Health Services.

   The community development philosophy needs to be actively discussed within the local health service so that the work of the Women's Health Team is received within a sympathetic framework.
5. Clarification of the campaigning role that is needed if services are to be more responsive. The team cannot have a realistic campaigning agenda within the NHS and so it will continue to work closely with the CHC and Health Campaign Unit (City Council). However, incidents of service failure will be fed back through the District Planning Group as women come in to contact with the team.
6. Responding to a demand for evening drop-in sessions. The monitoring of phone calls (very few records are kept except to help the team evaluate which issues are being raised by women) has indicated that many women in paid daytime work would value afterwork or evening openings.
7. Reviewing the pattern of work with women to see if the team is reaching

as many women as possible geographically, ethnically and across age groups. Active outreach work would be needed to make contact with women who may choose not to use the services to establish whether other forms of provision would be more appropriate.

8. Discussing the provision of health services for young women with the Health Promotion Unit (Senior Health Education Officer) (Education).

    Developing Well Women Centres or Clinics in communities where local women or community health workers have identified the need.

    Providing free childcare at all health services used by women (the community unit has successfully obtained funding for two years to employ creche workers for many community and hospital services).

    Creating better links with community colleges and further education so that women have the chance to become involved in courses and other activities.

    Prioritising work with black and ethnic minority women and challenging existing services to acknowledge the institutionalised racism inherent in the provision of health care.

9. Continuing the team's valuable national role with other women's health and community health initiatives. Consolidating the support links forged with North Manchester's community health projects, Salford Community Health Project and other community-based workers.

10. Reviewing women's health in the workplace and the need for cervical cytology provision with the Health Promotion Unit.

11. Ensuring that mental health is high on the team's agenda and rejecting the over-medicalisation of mental ill-health amongst women.

12. Promoting and publicising all services provided under the Well Women umbrella.

13. Planning more events that will reinforce the preventive health care aspects of the team's work.

14. Raising awareness of the health needs of informal carers.

15. Developing the existing skills of the workers through a commitment to on-going training.

The list of possible developments is endless and the Women's Health Team is only a small part of a network of women and other workers in community health projects throughout the country who are working in a similar way to challenge health inequalities and redress imbalance.

The future of all these initiatives looks increasingly bleak unless resources and commitment are forthcoming and the health needs of women are placed firmly at the top of the preventive health care agenda.

Reference

Orr, J. (ed.) (1987) *Health in the Community*. John Wiley, Chichester.

Part III

Changing Roles

Changing Ideas in Health Care
Edited by D. Seedhouse and A. Cribb
© 1989 John Wiley & Sons Ltd

Introduction to Part III

In order to achieve a common purpose between health services and other sectors, and to reduce the gap between professional and lay roles, it will be necessary for individuals from these different sectors to be able to meet each other in one-to-one transactions that take place under conditions of equality and mutual respect. This is why the aspirations of the health promotion movement to enable individual growth through personal, social, and environmental change are not limited to public health issues but reach into personal health care services.

The four chapters in Part III are all concerned with new forms of interaction in primary health care, they are all concerned in some sense with screening and prevention, and they all highlight the tensions that exist between professional and lay agendas, and the difficulty of striking a balance between them. They are drawn from primary health care because this is the area in which roles are already very broadly defined, and in which new ideas are having an impact. But as the earlier chapters have shown, there is no area of health care in which these issues do not arise.

The chapter by Brenda Spencer, Jane Morris and Helen Thomas is about a scheme that uses lay 'family workers' to provide social, psychological and practical support to pregnant women. Each woman in the scheme was assigned a particular family worker who performed a wide variety of functions, including helping with state benefits or re-housing, informal health education, or sometimes just listening and being there. The scheme is described as client-centred and holistic, and it is clear that these two principles are related. When clients are encouraged to determine their own needs and priorities for care or support it is inevitable that these will be diverse, and that they will cut across conventional expectations. Such a complex package of responsibilities could be seen as a radical reorientation of caring, but it might be better to see it, as the family workers tended to, as simply common sense plus common humanity. We all have some intuitive understanding of informal caring relationships, and of the needs for companionship, non-judgemental support and advice. The family workers were recruited and trained with this understanding in mind. Only when so many caring relationships have become formalised and professionalised do such ordinary (albeit precious) skills come to be seen as radical or esoteric.

The account highlights a number of the tensions that arise between the principles of the scheme and those of the health care system in which it was established and run. Indicative of these tensions was the insistence of the evaluation funders that the project's success should depend upon demonstrable improvements in birthweight. It is at best an oddity to assess a holistic project by a one-dimensional indicator, and this is apparent from the qualitative and process evaluations that are reported.

The discussion of the family worker scheme raises two issues that are central to changing roles in health care. Looking at pregnancy care in general the authors argue first that, 'little attempt is made to build on or even acknowledge lay competence', and second that considering the subjective needs of pregnant women, and 'the web of social disadvantage' faced by some, the high level of attention given to single risk factors, such as smoking, is of questionable value. In order to respect individuals, it is necessary to help them participate, to ensure that their role is not forced into some prescribed framework of categories and to acknowledge that there can be many concerns and activities of significance over and above the accepted medical priorities.

The conflict between focusing on specific risk factors and taking a broader, more responsive, approach is raised by the authors of the next two chapters. Elaine Fullard describes the overall aims and the first phases of the Oxford Prevention of Heart Attack and Stroke Project, in particular the new role of 'facilitators' to encourage screening and prevention in primary health care. Barbara Stilwell, who was one of the first nurse practitioners employed in Britain, presents a vivid account of her role in diary form. The former looks at the large practical task of setting up a population approach to screening and monitoring specific health indicators, with all of the financial, administrative and personnel ramifications. The latter looks at the day-to-day problems presented by actual individuals, problems that defy all but the broadest conceptions of health, and that cannot be met by a particular set of tasks, but only by sensitivity and imagination. In reality these two perspectives come together. Having a patient present for screening provides an opportunity to respond to other concerns, and vice versa. However, as both authors appreciate, there are considerable difficulties in combining reactive/caring and pro-active/ prevention roles in health care. It is usual for transactions to be defined in one way or the other, and for the other dimension to be lost because of the pressures of time and routine.

The first target of Fullard's project was to increase the level of identification, and recording, of risk factors for arterial disease. But in order to achieve even this comparatively modest objective it is necessary to develop the roles of receptionists and practice nurses to issue invitations for, and carry out, health checks. This creates a need to follow up some patients, and a demand from patients for more information about risk factors and symptoms. Also, the health checks provide scope for one-to-one health education, or counselling, or referral to further professional or lay help. It is in this way that a screening system built around specific risk factors has the potential to develop into a broad health promotion system. However, the greater the success the greater the difficulties of training and organisation, and the greater the problem of maintaining the motivation necessary for giving personal advice and support.

A facilitator's role is explained as being that of a catalyst, helping to initiate screening services in primary health care practices and providing continued support to ensure that practical problems do not create insuperable obstacles. The idea of planned and resourced facilitation is crucial to the success of all innovations. The speed with which this particular role (as well as the associated objectives) has spread, makes it a valuable model.

The idea behind the nurse practitioner role is that some people will find nurses more approachable than GPs, that nurses will be able to spend more time with patients (and so enable them to explore their concerns more), and that some pressure will be taken away from GPs. Stilwell's chapter puts the flesh on the bones of this idea. By providing a glimpse of the detail and the texture of the daily round the fact that health concerns do not come in tidy packages is made clear, as is the fact that there is little sense in distinguishing between personal or social problems and health problems. In Stilwell's voice there is the sound of a real divergence between the standard roles of health care workers and the reality of people's needs. There is also the sound of self-criticism and self-doubt; this is part of the price to be paid for giving up the security of technicalities, and the comforts of conventional roles and assumptions.

Stilwell expresses doubts about the value of screening unless it is backed up with good health education, and unless a better balance can be found between medical and non-medical interventions. One of the examples she gives is particularly instructive about the tension between coping with general problems and addressing specific risk factors. In the account of her home visit to a mother and daughter her reluctance to give the advice about weight control (advice that would be, on the face of it, appropriate) is made quite understandable.

Many of the issues raised by Stilwell are analysed in the final chapter of this collection, in which David Metcalfe discusses the theoretical and practical bases of teaching consultation skills. Like Stilwell he has a proper regard for the patients' own resources and competences, and he places great emphasis upon doctors becoming fully sensitive to the patients' interpretations and feelings. This is valued as a means of establishing trust, but equally as a condition of effectiveness. The alternative is to attempt to work with a partial grasp of the issues, and a partial use of the available data. However, the cost of taking this seriously, as Metcalfe sees, is to give up a position that is relatively secure both emotionally and in terms of personal power, and to expose oneself to a number of risks. The level of skill and understanding that is necessary in order to handle this delicate role can be achieved only with thorough and imaginative training. Without it Metcalfe believes there is little chance of strengthening clinical medicine.

Metcalfe's chapter pulls together a great many of the themes discussed elsewhere in this collection. His work shows that not only are equality, autonomy and holism central to health care, but also that it is possible to build the ideas and the practices appropriate to these themes into the education of health care professionals.

Changing Ideas in Health Care
Edited by D. Seedhouse and A. Cribb
© 1989 John Wiley & Sons Ltd

Chapter Ten
The South Manchester Family Worker Scheme

BRENDA SPENCER, JANE MORRIS AND HELEN THOMAS
Department of Epidemiology and Social Oncology
University of Manchester
UK

Introduction

This chapter documents our experiences in setting up and conducting a health promotion initiative, accompanied by a research programme, in the South Health District of Manchester, UK. The intervention consisted in the provision of 'family workers' to give social, psychological and practical support to women in pregnancy. The aim was to reduce stress and thereby improve the health and well-being of the women and their eventual offspring.

In describing the project, we also deal with a number of issues that are of relevance to a wider field of health promotion. The conceptual framework and principles that characterised the scheme involved the use of lay workers, and the adoption of a client-centred holistic approach. Problems were encountered with such an intervention linked to systems that are not based on the same principles. A recurrent theme of the intervention was that co-operation was crucial to its success. It was necessary to work with several different agencies with formal responsibility for the health and social welfare of the family workers' clients.

Another important aspect of the scheme was that the care provided by family workers was evaluated in the form of a randomised controlled trial. This meant reconciling a broad-based health promotion initiative with the risk factor approach of epidemiology. For more detail of this research, and the practical and ethical considerations associated with the scheme, refer to Spencer, *et al.* (1987).

Background to the Scheme

A government report on perinatal health, published in the UK (House of Commons Social Services Committee, 1980) highlighted widespread variations between different areas of the country. Birthweight is acknowledged as being one of the best indicators of perinatal health available (Chalmers, 1979) and, taking this indicator, Manchester compared badly with the country at large. In Manchester 10.2 per cent of all infants born weighed less than 2500 grams, compared with a figure of 7.3 per cent for England and Wales as a whole (Office of Population Censuses and Surveys, 1981a). It was these inequalities that prompted community physicians in the south of Manchester to look for new public health measures that might be taken to redress the balance.

The concept of the family worker comes originally from France. One author of this paper had spent time there studying maternal and child health care, and in particular the part played by the *'travailleuses familiales'* (Spencer, 1982). In France this service is nationally available through charitable organisations. Its original purpose was to 'replace' the mother in the home if for some reason she was unable to carry out her usual family and domestic responsibilities. Families usually contribute towards the cost of this help according to their income. However, in the department of Seine-Saint-Denis the *travailleuse familiale* was integrated into the public maternal and child health care service, so that pregnant women could be 'prescribed' a *travailleuse familiale* and therefore obtain help free of charge. The *travailleuse* was 'prescribed' for medical or practical reasons, such as to enable a mother of small children expecting another baby to obtain adequate rest, but was also able to intervene on other grounds, for example to provide social support to women who were particularly isolated, or were having difficulty coping. The *travailleuses familiales* frequently worked with socially disadvantaged families but emphasis was always placed on the need to take a non-judgemental approach and the importance of being 'at the same level' as the client.

Psychosocial stress has been pointed to as one mechanism by which social disadvantage may give rise to poor pregnancy outcome (Newton and Hunt, 1984; Newton *et al.*, 1979; Oakley, MacFarlane and Chalmers, 1982). Many factors are involved, some of which can be identified and could be acted upon. Factors often focused on are inadequate access to and uptake of services, poor access to information, physical effort, isolation, inappropriate diet, poor living conditions, ambivalence about the pregnancy and lack of local support (Brown and Harris, 1978; Hart, 1971; Martin, 1985; Papiernik, 1984; Spira *et al.*, 1981; Wolkind and Zajicek, 1981).

It was felt that while the health services may not be able to reverse the social disadvantage reflected in the perinatal statistics, it might at least be possible to compensate for it by the appropriate redirection of provision. This thinking led to the development of the family worker scheme, which aimed to provide social support to reduce stress and thereby improve the health of mothers-to-be and their babies.

Funding the Scheme

The workers themselves were funded by the Manpower Services Commission (MSC), which was a government-funded body designed to provide work experience for the long-term unemployed. Potential employers applied to the MSC for the salaries and expenses of workers on specific projects. In return employers provided staff training, basic office facilities and overall management and administration. The availability of these monies offered a tempting possibility to those wishing to introduce an innovation for which funding would not normally be available, particularly at a time of economic restraint. In this case it enabled us to set up a scheme with a certain amount of autonomy, yet within the National Health Service.

A certain common perspective was shared with the MSC in that our scheme was planned for a limited time period, and we were mainly employing and training older women with no formal qualifications, and hence limited employment prospects. However, the other aims of the scheme were not compatible with those of the MSC. For example, since we were attempting to offer continued support throughout pregnancy on an individual basis, it was important that the workers stayed for their full term of employment. Owing to their enjoyment of the work, they did tend to do this, but the official recommendation of the MSC was that sponsors should encourage staff to find permanent employment during rather than following their time on an MSC scheme.

Furthermore, the terms and conditions imposed by the MSC were subject to change at short notice. For example, we had understood that at the end of the first year (June 1982 to June 1983) we would be entitled to an extended year of funding if the scheme worked well. But towards the end of that time it emerged that although the scheme could continue only four of the 12 workers could be retained. The MSC made the condition that the rest had to be replaced by new staff. Naturally, the family workers did not find this acceptable and approached their trade union for support. According to agreements reached with the unions, the District Health Authority was able to conduct MSC schemes only if the approval of the relevant unions had been sought and obtained. Following the objections of the workers, the unions withheld their approval for the scheme to continue. The Health Authority were unable to obtain any concessions from the MSC and it was not until one year later, once the original workers had found satisfactory employment elsewhere, that the scheme was able to continue for a second year (Figure 1). However, we were at least able to double the number of workers employed and were fortunate enough to re-employ the original staff supervisor who provided a key element of continuity over the two years.

The Protocol Research

Since the family workers scheme was a new innovation in the UK, it was decided to devise it in a form that could be adequately evaluated. We wished to know whether the family workers would be successful in reducing stress and, in turn, whether this would be effective in improving birth outcome on a number of measures, chiefly birthweight and length of gestation. A research protocol to this effect was drawn up and submitted to the research committee of the Regional Health Authority. The evaluation was to be conducted in the form of a randomised controlled trial. In our original protocol we proposed that in addition to using clinical measures a psychologist be included in the

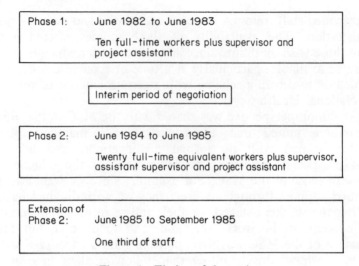

Figure 1   Timing of the project.

programme to assess the level of stress in the experimental and control groups and to relate this to pregnancy outcome. This component was specifically rejected by the committee. In our fourth submission to them, which was finally accepted, we were forced to concentrate solely on outcomes that could be measured in terms of clinical science. The emphasis thereby imposed on the evaluation was regretted: such a reductionist approach seemed at odds with the holistic concept of the project, and meant that in effect we had no way of examining the first part of our hypothesis regarding the improvement in maternal well-being. However, throughout the scheme we continued to attempt to obtain support from elsewhere to carry out a psychosocial assessment.

Organisation of the Scheme

The population covered by the trial was drawn from women booking in to have their babies at either of the two maternity units within the Health District. Since the role of the family worker was primarily one of prevention, any women booking in later than the 20th week of pregnancy were excluded. Asian women were excluded from the trial in view of the different birthweight distribution of these ethnic groups (Kurji and Edouard, 1984). Entry to the trial was also confined to those living within a certain geographical area. During the two periods of recruitment the notes of all women attending the booking-in clinics were screened.

In addition to the above conditions, a set of eligibility criteria were drawn up for entry to the trial. These criteria were mainly based on national statistics from the Office of Population Censuses and Surveys (1981b) and identified that part of the population most at risk of having a low birthweight baby. Table 1 summarises the criteria used. Any woman who satisfied at least two of these criteria was included. About two-thirds of those in the study satisfied

Table 1   Entry criteria

Age < 20 years

Underweight for height

Previous low birthweight baby(s) < 2500 grams

Parity = 0

Parity > 3

Marital status 'single'

Marital status common law

Previous spontaneous abortion(s) > 12 weeks
Previous perinatal death(s)
Previous infant death(s)

Social class IV or V (by husband's occupation)
Social class IV or V (by common-law husband's occupation
Single* woman, social class IV or V (by own occupation)†
Common-law woman, social class IV or V (by own occupation)†

Husband unemployed
Common-law husband unemployed
Single* woman unemployed
Common-law woman unemployed

Inter-pregnancy interval < 6 months

* Single includes widowed, separated and divorced women.
† In our study these two categories also include hairdressers, nursing auxiliaries and sales assistants. These occupations are coded other than IV or V by the Registrar General's Classification of Occupations (Office of Population Censuses and Surveys, 1980).

three or more criteria, although this would be expected since some criteria are interrelated; for example, women who were primiparous, less than 20 years old and unmarried.

On this basis, during any month of full recruitment approximately one-quarter of the women booking in were eligible for the trial. Following randomisation (see Figure 2) those in the experimental group were sent a letter containing a brief description of the scheme and a date and approximate time when the supervisor would call. In the second year we also included an illustrated leaflet (Figure 3). On her visit the supervisor explained the scheme in more detail, ascertained whether the woman was interested in having a family worker and, if so, which of the workers would be most appropriate.

We were able to recruit a total of 1288 women into the trial (Figure 4). Not all women who were offered a family worker accepted. Non-acceptance is a catchword used to denote the remainder of the experimental group other than those who received visits from a family worker. However, as can be seen from Table 2, this is not a homogeneous group. There were a number of reasons women did not, or were not able to, accept. The most common reason was that enough support was already available. 'Non-acceptance' should not be confused with some kind of drop-out rate. As far as the trial was concerned the 'treatment' consisted of the offer of a family worker, rather than in the actual assistance of one.

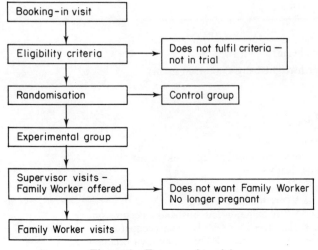

Figure 2   Entry to the trial.

Table 2   Reasons for non-acceptance

	Phase I	Phase II
Acceptors	40.1%	41.9%
Non-acceptors		
Well supported	19.2%	22.8 %
In employment	12.4%	4.0%
Moved away	10.2%	4.4%
Never at home	8.5%	15.9%
Not interested	6.8%	9.0%
No longer pregnant	2.8%	2.1%
Number in group	177	478

Ethical concern was expressed during the trial because women in the most acute need were not necessarily served by family workers. This concern arose firstly because the scientific nature of the trial required randomisation, thus excluding women who otherwise might have benefited. And secondly because the service was designed to prevent crises rather than to react to them.

The Role of the Family Worker

Prior to employment, our family workers had no formal professional training in the health or social services. They were, however, carefully selected according to personality and general life experience. A family worker had to be someone who was able to empathise easily without interfering in a client's life or allowing her to become over-dependent. Many, although not all, workers came from a broadly similar background to their clients and many had already brought up a family themselves.

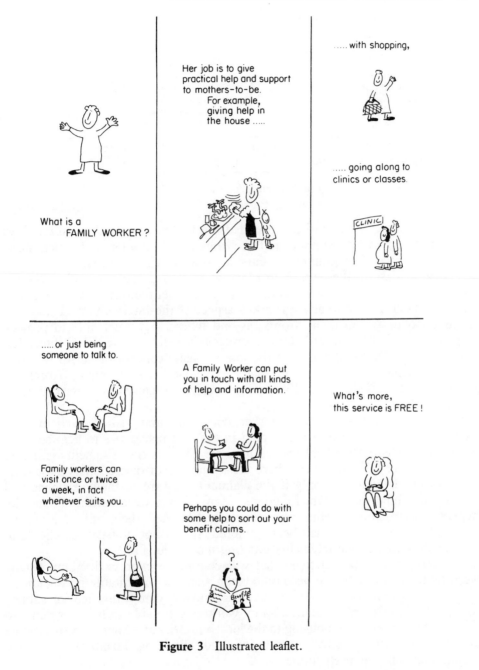

Figure 3   Illustrated leaflet.

At the start of the scheme workers attended a two-week induction course and had a brief training as appropriate, for example, most required familiarisation with making home visits and some in working with small children. Most training was, of necessity, conducted on an in-service basis. The work of the team was monitored by the supervisors, who held weekly or fortnightly interviews with each worker individually, in addition to maintaining regular

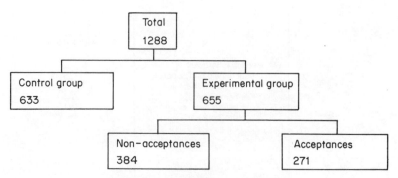

Figure 4 Participation in the trial.

telephone contact. All workers attended weekly meetings; these offered an opportunity for mutual support and exchange of information and experiences, and incorporated a programme of outside speakers and discussions.

The activities of the family workers were varied and depended on the individual needs of the client, as defined by the client and not by the worker. This client-centred approach was a key aspect of the intervention. They were called upon to act on many fronts, as and where they were able to provide help. This kind of health promotion corresponds well with the WHO 'lifestyles' approach (WHO, 1986) and with the more holistic concept of health which is currently being put forward in many areas (see, for example, Abraham, Hilgendorf and Welchman, 1983). The workers themselves described their work simply as 'common sense'.

Usually the first task for a worker when she first visited a client (and frequently the reason she was accepted in the first place) was to help sort out what state benefits the client was entitled to. The system of benefits is highly complex in the UK and, were there are a number of discretionary payments that can be claimed, but only if the claimant is aware of their existence and understands how the system functions. Many clients were entirely financially dependent on state benefits but had rarely obtained their full entitlement. Once all the possibilities had been explored, it was not unusual for clients to obtain additional single payments totalling more than £100.

Re-housing was another need that was commonly expressed. Many people were found to be living in accommodation that was unsuitable on a number of grounds. Living quarters might be overcrowded, damp, infested, or subject to repeated vandalism or theft. Family workers were able to help residents to present their cases for re-housing to the local authority and housing associations, and to help with removal, decoration and obtaining furniture once new accommodation had been found.

This role as intermediary applied to all services. Families were often suspicious, afraid or ignorant of authority. As far as possible, workers were there to reduce clients' fears and show them the way round the system rather than simply to take over on their behalf.

Domestic activity played less of a part in their work than we had originally led them to believe. When the workers began employment this had been emphasised as a way of conveying to the client that the family worker was not in a position of authority but was there to help 'at the same level'. One family worker achieved the ultimate assurance that she was doing her job correctly when she was told by a client 'I like you because you're common like me'!

Another aspect of the work was to accompany clients to antenatal clinics appointments or to classes, such as relaxation or parentcraft, which several would otherwise not have attended. The reaction of staff in the clinics was markedly different in the two hospitals. At one, the sister-in-charge felt that family workers offered an invaluable service and was welcoming and co-operative. This was in marked contrast to the reception received in the other clinic. Here, one or two staff who were opposed to the scheme even went so far as to humiliate workers in front of their clients. Reported incidents included the ejection of family workers from antenatal classes on the grounds that they had no right to be there and were therefore 'spying'. Yet, being constantly aware of the insecurity of the scheme's very existence, both supervisors and workers felt obliged to seek conciliation rather than challenge the actions of others. Furthermore, as lay temporary workers, they were not in a position to question the behaviour of established professionals.

For those clients with families already, childcare was an important part of the work, which sometimes involved showing women how to cope better with difficult children. They were able to time their visits to the most stressful parts of the day and help take or collect children to or from their school or nursery. The closeness of the relationship also enabled them to broach the subject of family planning. One major success was persuading a mother of nine to have sterilisation after the next baby. The mother's initial reaction to the suggestion had been that her husband 'wouldn't be bothered' to sign the consent form.

Health education was covered informally by, for example, shopping together. Budgeting was also a major problem for clients on a low income. Income was often insufficient to cover needs; in addition, a number of clients had succumbed to the temptation of hire-purchase offers or mail-order catalogues and found themselves in permanent debt.

Some women wanted a family worker simply for companionship. Asked at a meeting what were the necessary qualities to make a good family worker, those cited were 'good listener, keeps her prejudices to herself, common sense, streetwise, sensitivity, patience, compassion, sense of humour, adaptability and tolerance'. Initially, however, the workers required reassurance that they were doing their job when just listening. This was an aspect not always appreciated by NHS staff. One midwife remarked to a client, in front of a family worker, 'I wish I could get £70 a week for drinking tea'.

A number of community facilities were available in the area. Playgroups are one example, but clients were often unaware of, or hesitant about, using them. With family worker encouragement, they began to take advantage of these during pregnancy and it is hoped that they continued to do so after the worker left.

Qualitative Evaluation

In order to evaluate the scheme an extensive data set was developed, taken mainly from hospital medical records. This includes sociodemographic information, details of previous pregnancies, the course of the current pregnancy, the birth itself and birth outcome. In addition to these records, we attempted to conduct a six-month follow-up via the health visitors, whom we asked to complete a brief form on feeding practice, infant growth, need for and take-up of health services and an up-date on the social situation of the mother.

It is regrettable that we were not able to conduct a prospective psychological assessment along with the clinical assessment as we initially envisaged. Our experience indicates that we were in some measure able to relieve stress and improve maternal well-being, but if this does not translate clearly into the physiological outcome measures then there can be no quantifiable evidence of this. Following strenuous efforts to obtain funding from elsewhere to look at this aspect of the study, we were eventually able to establish collaboration with a research psychologist with separate financial support, who has conducted a one-year postnatal follow-up survey by postal questionnaire, using the Nottingham Health Profile (Hunt, McEwen and McKenna, 1985). Naturally, to include assessment of the women during their pregnancy would have been preferable.

Process Evaluation

The intervention was monitored in a number of different ways. It was important not only to be able to record the process taking place, but also to guide it. Qualitative material collected during the scheme included the supervisor's notes on each client taken from their regular interviews with the family workers, and feedback from the weekly group meetings. Towards the end of the scheme both the family workers and the supervisors drew up case study reports, and in addition completed questionnaires designed for them to assess the nature and outcome of their involvement with clients. This information, although indirect, indicated that the workers provided a high quality of care.

Clients often expressed their gratitude and several wrote letters of thanks. One, for example, wrote that her family worker 'does all my worrying for me which takes a lot of pressure from me so I can cope more'. Workers were invited to weddings and christenings and most attended at least one birth during the course of the scheme. They developed a strong sense of identity and great enthusiasm for the work and expressed a high level of job satisfaction.

An essential aspect of their work stemmed from their position as lay workers, which enabled them to identify with the client. In a longer-term project any tendency towards professionalisation should be avoided since this could totally deflect a scheme of this kind.

Co-operation with health service staff was at its best when the professionals saw that the family worker could offer more time and practical help than they were able to supply. This applied particularly to the social workers, with whom good teamwork was established. Liaison with other groups was more variable and depended to a large extent on the personal attitude of the individual professionals involved.

Some of the difficulties experienced can be attributed to the scheme's low priority relative to other health service activities. Often co-operation meant nothing more than tolerating our presence. One example of this was when we requested a 'liaison midwife'. Such an individual was identified to us, but it subsequently emerged that this midwife's day off was the same day as our weekly meeting and no further contact could be established.

At the start of the project we described the role of the family worker as one of primary prevention. Technically this was a possibility, since she visited from as early as possible in the pregnancy. However, from the clients' notes it is apparent that this term can only be used in a very limited sense. The history and total environment of some clients was such that any help from one individual could be no more than palliative, the web of social disadvantage being such that all problems compounded one another.

However, the scheme has at least served to highlight the needs of those most at risk, and the inadequacy of established services to respond to those needs. The implications of the Inverse Care Law (Hart, 1971) have long been a subject for debate. This law observes that those most in need of services are the least likely to take advantage of them, and vice versa. Hence, investment in services organised along traditional lines only serves to perpetuate inequality. Despite this knowledge pregnancy care remains strongly service-oriented and little attempt is made to build on or even acknowledge lay competence. Such resources as are available tend to focus on a medical approach to risk in pregnancy (for example, the increase in the use of ultrasound) despite the overwhelming evidence indicating the importance of social factors in determining pregnancy outcome.

Another common approach is the selection of individual risk factors for specific attention. The ultimate benefits of such an approach are questionable in view of the complex multi-factorial nature of risk. This approach rarely corresponds with the subjective needs of pregnant women, and indeed may sometimes conflict with those needs. Taking one of our clients as an example, it is a curious logic that would define a woman's problem as being that she smokes, when she lives in damp, overcrowded accommodation on a low income, and is depressed, single and expecting twins to a man married to someone else.

References

Abraham, F., Hilgendorf, L. and Welchman, R. (1983) The Tavistock Institute of Human Relations, Occasional Paper No. 7.

Brown, G. W. and Harris, T. (1978) *Social Origins of Depression: a Study of Psychiatric Disorder In Women*, pp. 270–293. Tavistock, London.

Chalmers, I. (1979) 'The Search for Indices', *Lancet*, 2, 17th November, 1063–1065.

Hart, J. T. (1971) 'Inverse Care Law', *Lancet*, 1, 27th February, 405–412.

House of Commons Social Services Committee (1980) *Perinatal and Neonatal Mortality*, Report 19 June 1980, HMSO, London.

Hunt, S. M., McEwen, J. and McKenna S. P. (1985) 'Measuring Health Status: a New Tool for Clinicians and Epidemiologists', *Journal of the Royal College of General Practitioners*, **35**, 185–188.

Kurji, K. H. and Edouard, L. (1984) 'Ethnic Difference in Pregnancy Outcome', *Public Health*, **98**, 205–208.

Martin, C. J. (1985) 'Stress in the Puerperium'. PhD Thesis, University of Manchester.

Newton, R. W., Webster, P. A. C., Binu, P. S., Maskrey, N. and Phillips, A. B. (1979) 'Psychosocial Stress in Pregnancy and its Relation to the Onset of Premature Labour', *British Medical Journal*, **2**, 411–413.

Newton, R. W. and Hunt, L. P. (1984) Psychosocial stress in pregnancy and its relation to low birthweight. *British Medical Journal*, **288**, 1191–1194.

Oakley, A., MacFarlane, A. and Chalmers, I. (1982) 'Social Class, Stress and Reproduction', in Rees, A. R., and Purcell, H. (eds) *Disease and the Environment*, pp. 11–50. John Wiley, Chichester.

Office of Population Censuses and Surveys (1980) *Classification of Occupations*. HMSO, London.

Office of Population Censuses and Surveys (1981a) *OPCS Monitor, Infant and Perinatal Mortality 1980*, DH3 81/3, October.

Office of Population Censuses and Surveys (1981b) *OPCS Monitor, Birthweight Statistics 1980*, DH3 81/4, November.

Papiernik, E. (1984) 'Prediction of the Preterm Baby', *Clinics in Obstetrics and Gynaecology*, **11**, 315–336.

Spencer, B. (1982) 'Family Workers in France', *Social Work Service*, No. 30, 4–8.

Spencer, B., Morris, J. and Thomas J. (1987) 'The South Manchester Family Worker Scheme', *Health Promotion*, **2**, No. 1, 29–38

Spira, N., Audras, F., Chapel, A., Debuisson, E., Jacquelin, J., Kirchhoffer, C., Lebrun, C. and Prudent C. (1981) 'Surveillance a domicile des grossesses pathologiques par les sages-femmes', *Journal de Gynecologie d'Obstetrique et de Biologie Reproductive*, **10**, 543–548.

Wolkind, S. and Zajicek, E. (eds) (1981) *Pregnancy: A Psychological and Social Study*. Academic Press, New York.

World Health Organization, Regional Office for Europe, Health Education Unit (1986) 'Lifestyles and Health'. *Social Science and Medicine*, **22**, 117–124.

Chapter Eleven
The Facilitator of Prevention in Primary Care: The Birth of a New Health Professional

ELAINE FULLARD
Oxford Prevention of Heart Attack and Stroke Project
Oxford Centre for Prevention in Primary Care
Radcliffe Infirmary
Oxford
UK

Introduction

'About a half of all strokes and a quarter of all the deaths from coronary heart disease in people under 70 are probably preventable by the application of existing knowledge.' This was the conclusion of the Royal College of General Practitioners' report on 'Prevention of Arterial Disease in General Practice' published in February 1981 (Royal College of General Practitioners, 1981). The challenge that now faces health professionals is to close the gap between what we know about reducing risk factors for heart disease, strokes and cancers and action. Much progress has been made in antenatal screening and child health care. The same energy, enthusiasm and systematic approach need to be applied to other age groups. Great Britain now has the unenviable record of having one of the highest rates of heart disease in the world, while other countries, such as the USA, Australia and Finland, have reduced their mortality rates due to heart disease by as much as 25 per cent in the last 20 years. Research into the top 20 causes of death in Oxfordshire show that heart disease, strokes and cancers are our major challenge (Figure 1).

The Oxford Prevention of Heart Attack and Stroke Project

What is needed is practical help for health professionals to enable them to apply more effectively existing medical knowledge about preventing heart disease. The emphasis of the Oxford project has been on the offer of practical

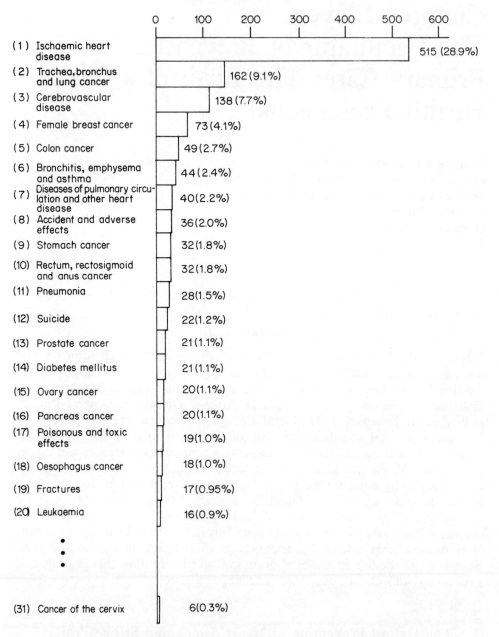

Figure 1   The top 20 causes of death in the Oxfordshire Health Authority 1986, age range 35–74 (OPCS, 1986) (men and women). (© 1988 E. M. Fullard, The Oxford Centre for Prevention in Primary Care, Radcliffe Infirmary, Oxford).

help and assistance to primary health care teams. The objectives of the project were as follows:

1. To demonstrate that it is possible for GPs and their teams to put into practice the recommendations of the Royal College of General Practitioners' (1981) report. The priority for action in men and women aged between 35 and 65 years is the identification of:
    High blood pressure,
    Smoking,
    Obesity.
2. To look at the contribution that a *facilitator* might have in helping primary health care teams to extend preventive medicine in general practice.
3. To produce a model that can be adopted widely.
4. To extend the collaboration between general practice, health authorities and family practitioner committees.

Method

Three experimental and three matched control group practices in Oxfordshire were chosen. The initial research project began in April 1982 and is now a permanent service funded by the health authority.

First audit

The medical records in the three experimental group practices were reviewed to obtain a baseline for information to establish the percentage of men and women aged 35–64 who had, in the preceding five years, a record of: (a) blood pressure measurement, (b) smoking habits, (c) an indication of obesity.

This audit was conducted with the permission of the GPs and with strict adherence to a protocol of confidentiality. An indication of obesity was used as a 'proxy' for raised lipids (i.e. raised levels of blood fats), and also as a visible target to highlight the need to encourage the population to reduce saturated fat intake.

The role of the facilitator

A facilitator is someone with a primary health care background, who literally, makes things easy or easier. He or she* is employed by the district health authority or family practitioner committee to offer help to interested practices in extending their preventive medicine (Fullard, 1987).

---

*As the majority of facilitators, nurses and receptionists connected with this project are women, the pronoun 'she' will be used throughout the rest of this chapter.

In order to raise the level of identification of the major risk factors for arterial disease, the facilitator encouraged the GPs to appoint a practice nurse to share the extra workload of screening their patients (Fullard, Fowler and Gray, 1984).

Facilitators act as cross-pollinators of good ideas to other practices that are considering starting a systematic approach to screening. The role includes:

1. Meeting the practice manager and receptionists, and, if needed, helping them to invite in the first few patients. The GP has an important role in encouraging and validating the invitation. The facilitator may suggest that every member of the team has a health check before the screening begins.
2. Providing a back-up service. For example, a facilitator has examples of health education literature, a supply of coloured height/weight charts as teaching aids for weight reduction, and examples of recall letters for mildly hypertensive patients.

The emphasis is on practical help, but to enable the facilitator to act as a temporary guest and informal adviser to the next interested practice, she does not carry out the clinical work herself. However, since most of the facilitators are nurses, should a screening nurse be off sick, the facilitator can, with the practice's permission, help out by conducting a clinic.

The method of screening

Patients in the target age group who attend the practice for any reason are invited by the receptionist to see the nurse for a brief health check (subsequently nicknamed 'a human MOT'). This avoids both the time and cost of sending postal invitations. Some nurses offer clinics in the mornings and evenings to meet the needs of the working population. This 'opportunistic' approach can reach 75 per cent of a practice population within a year and 90 per cent within five years.

Health checks take about 20 minutes and are either organised in special sessions by the nurse in health-check clinics or interspersed with her other treatment-room work. The nurse asks about relevant family history and diabetes, records blood pressure, measures weight and height, enquires about diet, smoking, alcohol and, when appropriate, oral contraception (Figure 2). Blood pressure measurement and the subsequent course of action follow a protocol (Figure 3) and smoking and dietary advice is given in accordance with guidelines (Astrop, Fullard and O'Dwyer, 1985).

Blood lipids (that is, blood fats) are measured selectively, only in those with a personal or family history of coronary heart disease at or below the age of 55 and in patients with multiple risk factors. Tests for blood sugar are only carried out in those who are seriously obese (more than 30 per cent overweight) or who have a family history of diabetes.

Information is recorded in the notes on a special health summary card (Figure 2) and the outside of the patient's records are labelled with the date for next review (Fullard et al., 1984).

HEALTH SUMMARY   FEMALE

Name [   ]   D.O.B. [   ]

SMWD [   ]   No. [   ]

Own Occupation
and
Partner's Occupation [   ]

| Date 1st B/P [   ] | Date 2nd B/P [   ] | Date 3rd B/P [   ] | Mean if applicable [   ] | Notes |

Height [   ]   Weight [   ]   Ideal Weight [   ]

Nutrition Advice [   ]   Exercise [   ]

| Smoker | | Cigarettes | | Pipe | | Since 19 | |
| Non Smoker | | Never | | Stopped 19 | | | |

Family History of CVA or MI [   ]

| Diabetes | Yes | | Insulin | | OHD | | Diet | |
| | No | | | | | | | |

| Oral Contraception Years of Use | Current | | Past | | Never | |

| Last Cervical Smear | Date | | Result | |

| Rubella | Immune | Yes | | No | | Date | |
| | Vaccination | Yes | | No | | Date | |

| Date of Tetanus | 1st | | 2nd | | 3rd | | Booster | |

| Urine | Date | | Protein | | Sugar | |

| Alcohol | |

Notes / Advice given / Further action

CONTINUATION

Date	B/P	Smoking	Weight	Contraceptive Change	Rubella	Tetanus	Cervical Smear		

Figure 2   Health summary. (Reproduced from Fullard *et al.* (1987) by permission of the *British Medical Journal*.)

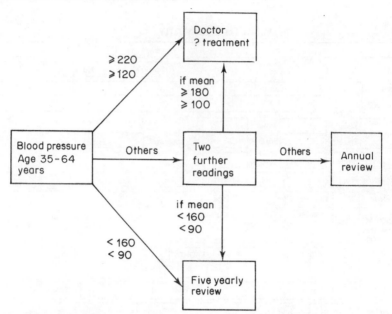

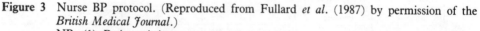

Figure 3   Nurse BP protocol. (Reproduced from Fullard *et al.* (1987) by permission of the *British Medical Journal*.)
NB: (1) Patient sitting;
    (2) Note fear/anxiety/anger/cold, if present;
    (3) ? Empty bladder;
    (4) ? Adequate cuff to encircle arm;
    (5) Rate of fall of pressure 2 mmHg per second;
    (6) Record to nearest 2 mmHg;
    (7) DBP Phase V (complete absence of sound) unless this = zero., then use Phase IV (muffling) and record 'IV' after recording in medical notes.

Second audit

The second review of the medical records was made $2\frac{1}{2}$ years later to establish whether, with the help of a facilitator, the general practitioners and nurses had been able to raise the level of identification of risk factors for arterial disease in the age group. Since this project was initially funded for only three years, the project team's aims were not to look at whether there had been a decrease in the number of strokes and heart attacks. Although this would have been valuable and satisfying it was not investigated because the numbers in the populations studied were too small and the time-span too short for significant alterations to be likely. The research team relied, too, on the strong evidence from larger epidemiological trials with longer intervention and follow-up programmes, which have shown that controlling hypertension does reduce the incidence of strokes (Australian National Blood Pressure Study Management Committee 1980; Helgeland, 1980; Hypertension Detection and Follow-up Co-operative Group, 1979).

The Oxford project aimed to make the first step of putting preventive medicine into practice. About 50 per cent of hypertensive people do not know that they have high blood pressure, neither do their doctors, and many have never been asked about their smoking habits. Help cannot be initiated if these risk factors are unknown. Naturally, there was concern about the management of patients once risk factors had been identified. Advice about smoking cessation, weight loss and anti-hypertensive therapy was provided by the GPs and nurses involved.

The ideal aim is for 100 per cent of patients aged 35–64 to have these risk factors identified, then, once this most vulnerable group has been screened, to extend the age group to include everyone from 20 years upwards.

Results

There was a team effort by the GPs and their nurses to identify risk factors.

Initially, blood pressure was recorded in 35 per cent of the medical notes in the intervention practices (compared with 37 per cent in controls); smoking habits in 11 per cent in intervention practices (compared with 12 per cent in controls); and weight or an indication of obesity in 12 per cent in intervention practices (compared with 13 per cent in controls). The differences between intervention and control practices were not significant, indicating that they were well matched. However, the final audit showed that although there were substantial increases in the recording of blood pressure, smoking habits and weight in all practices, this was much greater in the intervention practices than it was in the controls.

After the $2\frac{1}{2}$ year interval, 59 per cent of records in intervention practices had a blood pressure recording (compared with 49 per cent in controls), 49 per cent a mention of smoking habit (compared with 21 per cent in controls) and 45 per cent measurement of weight (compared with 19 per cent in controls). Numerically, in the three intervention practices, 1022 more people had had their blood pressure recorded, 2327 more had had their smoking habits recorded and 2158 more had had their weight recorded than in the three control practices (Figure 4). Eighty-four patients with sustained blood pressure readings at or above 180/100 were identified, including three patients with sustained measurements greater than 220/120.

Thus, the introduction into intervention practices of a systematic case-finding approach, using practice nurses to conduct health checks and with the help of a facilitator, as an informal adviser/resource agent and trainer, substantially enhances ascertainment of risk factors. Increase in blood pressure recordings was doubled, the increase in recording smoking habits quadrupled and weight recording increased more than five-fold in the intervention practices compared with the controls (Fullard, Fowler and Gray, 1987). General practitioners incurred some extra costs by extending the number of practice nurse hours but these were modest (see Figure 5). Equally, extra work for doctors is generated by detection of hypertensive patients needing treatment, but few would deny the value of this. The nurses are responsible for recalling the borderline hypertensive patients. These patients accounted for 82 per cent of

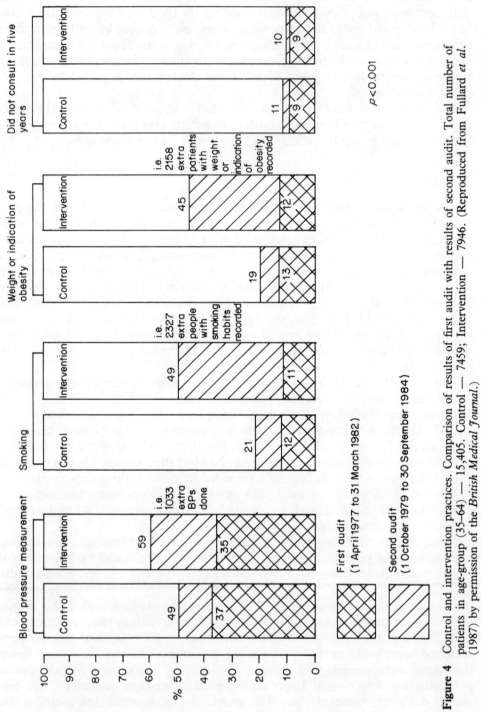

Figure 4 Control and intervention practices. Comparison of results of first audit with results of second audit. Total number of patients in age-group (35–64) — 15,405. Control — 7459; Intervention — 7946. (Reproduced from Fullard et al. (1987) by permission of the *British Medical Journal*.)

Sharing the Workload

Cost

Nursing Sister Grade 'G' — 10 hours per week

£6.65 per hour	=	£66.50 per week
Less FPC 70% reimbursement	=	£19.95
Less 40% tax relief on remaining 30%	=	£11.97
Therefore, net cost to practice	=	£11.97

Items of service fees (FPC)

New rates as from 1 April 1988 – Gross and net fees

Fee for cervical smear	£8.20 (less tax)	=	£4.92
First and second tetanus injections	£2.80 (less tax)	=	£1.68
Third tetanus and booster injections	£4.10	=	£2.46

Therefore, practice nurse employed for 10 hours
at £11.97 per week would need to do

one overdue cervical smear	=	£4.92
and three tetanus boosters	=	£7.38
to more than equal the salary costs to the practice		
Total	=	£12.30

Figure 5   Sharing the workload.

the newly diagnosed hypertension. For the practice nurse this new extended role is challenging and satisfying. She becomes a full professional partner in the primary care team. Although health visitors can do the job, in many situations they are too busy to take on this additional work.

It appears that it is the *practical problems* of getting a screening programme organised and running that deter primary health care teams. General practitioners made the following remarks about the *facilitator help* and the screening programme:

'It's the best thing that's happened to the practice.'
'We are doing the obvious, we should have done this before, we just needed someone to get us organised and give us a bit of help.'
'We just needed a "kick" to get us going!'
'I feel it is a team effort. It has crystallized what we have been trying to do.'

(The Oxford Prevention of Heart Attack and Stroke Project, 1987)

The *audits* of the medical records have highlighted the need for a much more systematic approach to screening and counselling about risk factors. The MRC trial on mild hypertension (Medical Research Council Working Party, 1985) indicated, for example, how much more 'at-risk' smokers are than non-smokers, and yet audits show that many patients on anti-hypertensive treatment have not been asked about their smoking habits (Stern, 1986). Similarly, the need to try non-pharmacological ways of reducing blood pressure levels, by reducing obesity and alcohol intake, if excessive, is not matched in the degree to which these risk factors are recorded (Fullard et al., 1984).

How Does the Oxford Project Fit in with Other Systems of Care?

The facilitator's role is to act as a catalyst and practical helper to primary health care teams. These teams are an important yet small cog in the very large wheel of health promotion. However, by their contact with the public, they are in a key position to encourage people to use and benefit from other services.

Information about risk factors, nevertheless, needs to be made relevant to individuals. Members of the team have a golden opportunity to do this. During health checks there is the scope for one-to-one health education, the answering of queries, and the translation of the mass media message to what it means for that particular patient in terms of lifestyle changes.

The high response rate to the invitation by the receptionists in the Oxford project (only 3 per cent of the first 4000 patients screened definitely declined the invitation) and the enthusiasm of the public for this new kind of caring reflects the public's awareness of the need for preventive medicine. Wallace and Haines (1984) found that patients expect to be counselled on their health behaviour.

The practice nurse in the health check can use her other colleagues as resources. For example she might involve the community dietitian. Further examples are:

1. Referral to the general practitioner for help from the Social Services.
2. Referral to a marriage guidance counsellor.
3. Sharing information about community provision of exercise classes, slimming groups, stop-smoking groups, and relaxation classes.

Local group leaders can issue the practice nurse with details of times and dates of classes so that she can promote these opportunities for exercise and care.

What Do the Patients Say?

Patients have greatly welcomed these health checks and have made the following observations:

> 'I think it's a marvellous idea, the NHS should have been doing this a long time ago.'
> 'Yes, I should be very pleased to have my blood pressure checked. I do have a check at work but I should like my family doctor to have it on his records.'

'I found the booklets very interesting.' [The Health Education Authority's publication on 'Guide to Healthy Eating' and 'Beating Heart Disease' are given to the patients by the nurse.]
'I am unemployed, so would miss out on check-ups at work.'
'I'm glad the men are not being forgotten, my wife always seems to be the one who gets all the attention.'

(Oxford Prevention of Heart Attack and Stroke Project, 1987)

Since women consult their general practitioners twice as often as men, and men are more at risk from heart disease, wives are being encouraged to ask their husbands to make an appointment. Several couples come in together to see the nurse.

A questionnaire was sent out to all of the first 2000 patients to have a health check. Results showed that the majority of patients found the health checks reassuring and did not mind seeing the nurse instead of the doctor. But they wanted more information about risk factors, and, in particular, early symptoms of cancer. 19 per cent of 35–49-year-olds had difficulty attending the clinics at the times offered (Anderson, 1986). Therefore, primary care teams need to provide clinics to fit in with their clients' needs.

Benefits to the Practice

The facilitator first helps the receptionist invite a few patients for the health check. But it is a team effort, and much of its success is probably due to the vital role of the receptionist in her initial invitation. The receptionists have felt involved and enjoy the overwhelmingly positive reaction of the patients. Receptionists have commented:

'I think it shows concern by the practice.'
'I enjoy asking people, as it is nice to offer something rather than saying I'm sorry, there are very few appointments left.'
'The men are proud as Punch when they have been back to see the nurse having lost weight and their blood pressure has dropped.'
'It is extra work at first, but well worthwhile I think.'

(Oxford Prevention of Heart Attack and Stroke Project, 1987)

What Are the Problems?

These can be divided into three categories: 1. Training needs; 2. Organisation; 3. Maintaining motivation.

1. Training needs

When a practice nurse changes from her traditional role to include health promotion in her work, extra skills are sometimes necessary. At present, there is relatively little structured training for practice nurses and although many

English National Board courses are now available, the amount of time devoted to preventive medicine is not always sufficient. For example, before embarking on a screening programme, refresher training on the need for taking accurate blood pressure measurements is sometimes needed. It is also essential that the practice has an agreed policy of everyone reading blood pressures to Phase V (complete absence of sound). Similarly, sphygmomanometers need to be checked for accuracy and cuffs of different sizes need to be available for each GP and nurse.

The facilitator can act in a similar role to a clinical nurse tutor in teaching the practice nurses in her district, and can also refer them to specialist courses in hypertension screening.

2. Organisation

Lack of time and extra workload are two commonly quoted problems. The problem of lack of time can either be solved by the existing practice nurse taking on extra hours or by employing a nurse for a few extra hours per week (See Figure 5) to provide protected time for the screening. The facilitator can help in all the initial organisation of setting up the screening clinic as indicated in the section on 'the role of the facilitator'.

Since the nurse is responsible for the follow-up of any newly diagnosed mildly hypertensive patients and recalls patients needing extra counselling about diet and smoking, the GPs have not noticed the extra workload. The GP, nevertheless, has an ideal opportunity to reinforce and follow up the advice that the nurse has given in her 'human MOT' clinics, since she highlights risk factors on a summary card that is filed in the front of the medical records (see Figure 2).

3. Maintaining motivation

Practice teams often enjoy an initial period of enthusiasm, full clinics and patients telephoning for appointments. However, prevention can very easily get 'pushed out' by other demands. For example, since the recall time for cervical smears is now three years in many areas, the 'humdrum' business of helping and advising people about their smoking and dietary habits can get forgotten. Personal contact has been found to be a strong factor in overcoming barriers to change (Horder, Bosanquet and Stocking, 1986) and since the facilitator's work is practice-based, she can help practices to establish ways for teams to monitor their own successes or failures in their screening programmes.

The district facilitator may be able to offer a 'Rent-an-Audit' team. The Oxfordshire team consists of two trained auditors who work to a protocol of strict confidentiality for the patients and the practice. These professionals may be hired by a practice for a small charge and can usually conduct an audit in two or three afternoons with minimal disturbances to the practice (Gray, O'Dwyer, Fullard and Fowler, 1987).

Evaluation of the numbers of patients seen and risk factors that have been identified can be made by keeping a *log book* that involves little clerical work.

The log book (Figure 6) can give an indication to the team of the gender and age-group of patients attending the health checks, the number who do not arrive, women with overdue smears, and referral rates for tetanus boosters, hypertension and cholesterol tests. In addition, the log book gives a good excuse for the team to celebrate significant events, such as when the hundredth patient has been screened. Presentation of *case studies* at practice meetings maintains enthusiasm and interest in the programme. Evaluation of *recall* for newly diagnosed hypertensive patients, by maintaining a card index register in a box file or by registering recalls on a computer, are ways of ensuring that risk factors are followed up.

Finally, and most important of all, *the patients' needs, expectations and experience* of the screening programme can be measured. An anonymous questionnaire could be returned by a sample of patients. This questionnaire would need to be completed by those declining as well as those accepting the invitation. Informal verbal feedback is useful and a little positive feedback from patients encourages the team enormously.

A team can derive great job satisfaction from the feeling that, through the use of an organised approach to screening their population, they are 'on top of the problem'.

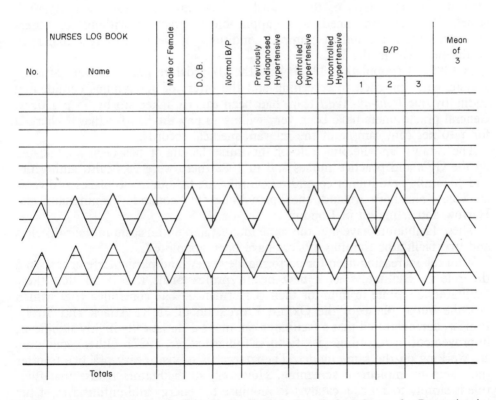

Figure 6 Nurse's log book.(© 1983 E. M. Fullard, The Oxford Centre for Prevention in Primary Care, Radcliffe Infirmary, Oxford.)

Where Do We Go from Here? A Look at Future Training

The rapid adoption of health screening and the equally rapid development of the practice nurse will further press the case for a formal post-basic training such as health visitors and district nurses now enjoy. This growth may well move in tandem with the development of the nurse practitioner concept.

A concern by GPs to include communication skills has been noticeable in training schemes. It is to be hoped that the same attention will be focused on nurse training. An increasing awareness is now needed for general practices to regard their patients in population terms and to set priorities for action to tackle the most prevalent diseases demonstrated in the top 20 causes of death in a district (see Figure 1). It is high time to devote as much energy and resources into counselling women about the need to change dietary and smoking habits and to screen for blood pressure as has been devoted to screening for cervical cancer.

As an even higher priority it is time to focus attention on the higher early mortality figure for males, to ensure that screening for men is provided as well as for women.

The Future of the Facilitator

One of the main aims of the Oxford project was to produce a *transferable model*. This screening needs to be applicable to practices without computers or age/sex registers, and in cramped conditions, if we are to effect change in all the practices in the UK.

In 1988, 51 (population 383,944) of the Oxfordshire practices were offering a systematic approach to screening and the offers of anonymous confidential audits by our *Rent-an-Audit* team had been eagerly taken up by 55 practices. General practitioners have been very willing to pay the £15 fee that is charged for a 10 per cent sample of the relevant medical records.

The catalyst and helping role of the nurse facilitator has been appreciated by the GP's and practice nurses and in 1988 there were 53 health authorities and 20 family practitioner committees employing facilitators in places as diverse as Wales, Northern Ireland, the Forth Valley in Scotland, Birmingham, and Harrow and Islington in London.

These facilitators have met the same interest and enthusiasm in their districts and two facilitator training officers have been appointed.

With the increasing need for performance review and particularly in assessing the role of facilitators as a new health professional, it is vital that these facilitators continue to monitor their performance. The controlled trial, which was the initial phase of the Oxford Prevention of Heart Attack and Stroke Project, demonstrated that a facilitator can make a statistically highly significant improvement in recording risk factors (Fullard et al., 1987). Other facilitators are working on the same model. Their target is to visit every practice to offer their help to implement screening. However, all facilitators realise that their role is simply to act as a catalyst to mobilise the energy and enthusiasm of the army of primary health care teams to tackle the epidemic of arterial disease.

References

Anderson, R. (1986) 'Results of Questionnaire on Patients' Attitudes to Health Checks'. Personal communication.

Astrop, P. J., Fullard, E. M., and O'Dwyer, M. A. (1985) 'Nurses Guidelines', The Oxford Prevention of Heart Attack and Stroke Project (unpublished).

Australian National Blood Pressure Study Management Committee (1980) 'The Australian Therapeutic Trial in Mild Hypertension', *Lancet*, **i**, 1261–1267.

Fullard, E. M. (1987) *First in the Field. Community View*. Smith & Nephew, London.

Fullard, E. M., Fowler, G. H., Gray, J. A. M. (1984) 'Facilitating Prevention in Primary Care', *British Medical Journal*, **298**, 1582–1587.

Fullard, E. M., Fowler, G. H., Gray, J. A. M. (1987) 'Promoting Prevention in Primary Care: a Controlled Trial of Low Technology, Low Cost Approach', *British Medical Journal*, **294**, 1080–1082.

Gray, J. A. M., O'Dwyer, M. A., Fullard, E. M. and Fowler, G. H. (1987) 'Rent-an-audit — Letters', *Journal of the Royal College of General Practitioners*, **37**, 177.

Helgeland, A. (1980) 'Treatment of Mild Hypertension: a Five-year Controlled Drug Trial. The Oslo Study', *American Journal of Medicine*, **60**, 725–732.

Horder, J., Bosanquet, N. and Stocking, B. (1986) 'Ways of Influencing the Behaviour of General Practitioners', *Journal of the Royal College of General Practitioners*, **36**, 517–521.

Hypertension Detection and Follow-up Co-operative Group (1979) 'Five-year Findings of the Hypertension Detection and Follow-up Programme: Reduction in Mortality of Persons with High Blood Pressure, Including Mild Hypertension', *Journal of the American Medical Association*, **242**, 2562–2571.

Medical Research Council Working Party, 1985 'MRC Trial of Treatment of Mild Hypertension: Principal Results', *British Medical Journal*, **291**, 97–104.

Office of Population Censuses and Surveys (1986). 'The Top Twenty Causes of Death in the Oxfordshire Health Authority, 1986, Age Range 35–74 (Men and Women), Extracted from OPCS, VS3. Returns. OPCS, London.

Open University (1987) 'What's Being Done?' *Coronary Heart Disease: Reducing the Risk*, Chapter 4. Open University Press, Milton Keynes.

Oxford Prevention of Heart Attack and Stroke Project. Progress Report April 1982 to April 1987 (unpublished). The Oxford Centre for Prevention in Primary Care, Oxford OX2 6HE.

Royal College of General Practitioners (1981) *Prevention of Arterial Disease in General Practice. Report from General Practice No. 19*, RGGP, London.

Stern, D. (1986) 'Management of Hypertension in Twelve Oxfordshire General Practices', *Journal of the Rogal College of General Practitioners*, **36**, 549–551.

Wallace, P. G. and Haines, A. P. (1984) 'General Practitioners and Health Promotion: What Patients Think', *British Medical Journal*, **289**, 534–536.

Chapter Twelve
Diary of a Nurse Practitioner

BARBARA STILWELL
Department of Nursing
King's College
London
UK

There is now a Nurse Practitioner working in this surgery. She is a trained Nurse and Health Visitor with extra training in recognising and advising on common family health problems. If you would like to see the Nurse Practitioner please tell the Receptionist.★

Monday

The Monday morning waiting room is always full. Pressure on emergency appointments is greater than on other days so the nurse practitioner seems to be a good alternative to consulting nobody, even for those patients who say that when they go to the doctors it's the doctor they want to see. Two people this morning might have felt they had no choice *but* to see the nurse practitioner. The first was Mr Lymes.

A message came from the receptionist that a man was shouting the odds in the waiting room about the length of time he has been waiting. I've been seeing patients for 2 1/2 hours and instinctively feel less than sympathetic. Perhaps the patient has been waiting that long too.

I go to fetch him from the waiting room. The doctors here use buzzers to indicate to the receptionist that they are ready for the next patient, and she sends them in. I feel happier meeting and greeting people who come to see me, but maybe it does take longer and increases waiting time. Mr Lymes is a tall, heavy and extremely angry West Indian man.

It is perhaps, slightly unusual for patients to be angry with doctors or nurses. They prefer to make their complaints and vent their wrath on long-suffering receptionists, and anyone else in the waiting room who can hear.

★This notice explained to patients the presence of a nurse practitioner in an inner city general practice from 1982 to 1985. The whole project was evaluated in terms of the patients' attitudes to the role, the style and content of the nurse practitioner's work and acceptibility of the role to her colleagues.

Mr Lymes sits uneasily in his chair, looking as though he is about to explode. 'You seem to be angry' I say, to allow him to admit to his feelings. He tells me about his waiting time, and that I was the only person he could see. 'I don't think you can help me,' he says. A consultation with the nurse practitioner is meant to be a real choice rather than Hobson's choice. I tell him I'm sorry, and say that I'll arrange for him to see the doctor, but maybe he'd like to tell me about the problem since he's here. He is worried, he says, that he has a sexually transmitted disease and that he and his live-in girlfriend need treatment.

He has had sex outside this stable relationship and says 'I just want you to make me clean'. We talk at length about which part of him we would like cleansed; we eventually conclude that it could be his conscience. Nevertheless, I ask a male doctor colleague to examine Mr Lymes (he finds nothing abnormal) and I arrange to see Mr Lymes's girlfriend soon. He has been with me for half an hour. His anger has gone now, and he tells me that I have helped him. 'What is your name, so I can ask for you next time?'

In the afternoon Mr Lymes's girlfriend turns up. He has sent her to get treatment for an infection which he says she gave to him. I ask about their relationship and she says it's not good lately; he stays out more and seems to have lost interest in their daughter. I wonder how she copes in their flat, alone with a three-year-old for most of the day, living on social security and with no prospect of a job in this depressed inner city area. I take a swab from her vagina and a cervical smear. All looks well, so we talk more about her life and its frustrations. I invite her to come and see me again if she needs to talk things over. I have nothing to offer. I have only my listening skills, and I feel inadequate to help her.

Confidentiality is essential for this job, but still I feel frustrated that Mr Lymes is blaming his steady girlfriend for his supposed infection, when he and I know that he acquired the fear of it elsewhere.

The second patient who saw me today, although she had hoped to see the doctor, was a young woman, Clare, who had pain on urinating. When I fetched Clare from the waiting room she was brisk and possibly rather brusque. We sat down in my room in chairs carefully placed (by me) at the corner of my desk — an effective collaborative position, the psychologists tell us. Clare said 'Do you mind if I move the chairs back? I feel too close to you.' I was surprised and somewhat discomfited that my carefully learned theory was not, in this case, effective. As I looked at Clare's notes I saw that she had a history of mental illness, once diagnosed as schizophrenia. There, I thought, is the problem — it's her mental instability, not my theory, or is it?

How easy it is to label people. Once that label is written in the person's medical notes, it becomes 'official' and it is no longer necessary to take that person seriously. It is also easy to imagine that such labelling behaviour is practised by someone else, never by me. I should have learned this lesson long ago, when I was consulted by a young woman who complained of feeling anxious, tired and weak. I read in her notes that she had for many years taken tranquillisers, having consulted her doctor for a series of 'neurotic disorders'. At the time I was new at the job of nurse practitioner. This meant in my case that I was inclined to believe the medical notes and attribute the present symptoms to anxiety, but it also meant that I carried out a very thorough physical examination. What I found was a dangerously high blood pressure, so severe that immediate hospital admission was necessary. In the light of that experience Clare deserved some kinder reaction to her request to move the chairs: theories should be there to be adapted to people's needs.

Tuesday

Today we invite people over 60 to come to the surgery for a health check. Each person sees a doctor, the nurse practitioner, the practice nurse, and the social worker and a dental therapist. Their physical, mental, emotional and social conditions are assessed by this team and they are given appropriate advice or help.

It's a service that most practices don't offer, and one that the senior partner here began. Most people attending are glad to be asked and to have the opportunity of asking questions themselves.

It is normally assumed by health professionals that the screening of a well population for factors that may eventually produce disease can only be a good thing. By and large I expect they are right, but I wonder whether enough information is always given to the person being screened, on the nature of the risk factor discovered, the chances of its producing some serious illness in the future and the options open for treatment?

Taking patients' blood pressure is *de rigeur* these days, since hypertension is known to cause heart disease and strokes. But the treatment of hypertension is a complicated business. It sometimes involves medication, but it can also include advice to lose weight, exercise programmes, and the reduction of dietary fat. Stress control may also be indicated. Do health professionals always ensure they can offer alternatives or adjuncts to medication when screening for hypertension? Since one of the purposes of nurse practitioner care is health education, I feel reasonably happy that I can offer non-medication help with the control of risk factors, and I like to believe I am honest with the people who consult me. A recent addition to our screening routine has made me less confident about my commitment to honesty with patients. We have introduced a questionnaire to screen patients for senile dementia. This is thought to be a problem that may be hidden from the GP. Relatives have been known to cope with the effects of a dementing elderly parent until the problem overwhelms them.

I find it difficult to say to people who appear to be mentally perfectly normal: 'I'd like to ask you some questions now to see if you are becoming demented'. Instead I use some euphemism, such as 'Can I ask you some questions to see if you are getting more forgetful?' The questions themselves are embarrassing:

'Where do you live?'
'Who is the present Sovereign?'

'When did the Second World War start?'
'Can you count backwards from 20 to 1?'

It's like a school test; is it demeaning to these elderly people?

Sometimes I alter the words or phrases if I think people won't understand —
there are many elderly people in this area who left school aged 12. Instead of
'Who is the present Sovereign?', I say 'Who is on the throne?' and am not
taking the test entirely seriously.

I wonder if the results of the tests are valid. Maybe I'm sending home
hundreds of dementing elderly people to leave the gas on or wander their
neighbourhood after dark?

I ask my colleagues about the test. One says that when she administers it
she doesn't say what it is for. The other doesn't worry about it at all. Is it
right, I wonder, to tell 'white lies' when to tell the truth might cause problems
that could be avoided? Notwithstanding this questionnaire, today I feel I've
helped someone.

An 86-year-old man came for screening today. I asked him if there was
anything particular I could help him with. He told me he had no relatives,
and was concerned about . . . Here, his voice faltered, so I prompted him
'about . . .?' 'Well,' he said, 'You know . . . after I die . . .'. The man literally
had *not one* living relative, and was, as he put it, worried about 'the disposal
of the dead' — in other words, his funeral arrangements. I was not sure what
he should do, but with the man's consent I contacted local solicitors who gave
us advice.

A few days later he came back to see me to collect a booklet I'd ordered
for him called 'What to do when someone dies'. He was cheerful and seemed
relieved to be sorting out this problem. He had come for general health
screening, which is a check on physical, emotional, mental and social status.

Wednesday

This morning was one of high drama. In the middle of my consulting time
another nurse in the practice opened my door to say 'I'd value your opinion
about someone who has been taken ill in the waiting room'. I replied 'Right-
oh, I'll be with you in a minute.' She said just one word in reply: 'Now'. In
the waiting room was a lady in her sixties, not known to me. She was blue
and apparently having a seizure. I checked her pulse and found that she had
suffered a cardiac arrest. The waiting room was full.

Together, my colleague and I tried to lift, but in fact dragged, the rather
heavy lady into a treatment room, where we began resuscitation immediately.
The nurse went to get two of our medical colleagues and between us we
continued cardiac massage and artificial respiration for 20 minutes. At one
point we set up an ECG machine and I took off the woman's boots. As I did
so I had the sudden realisation that this wasn't a patient but a *person* that we
were 'working on'. We failed in our attempts and the woman, who, it
transpired, had had a long history of heart disease, died on the floor of our
treatment room at 10.30 a.m. According to her neighbour she had been awake

with chest pains since 5 a.m. but hadn't wanted to bother the doctor. Her boots had obviously been her best — well kept and newish — and her clothes were her best too — worn especially to see the doctor — a big occasion for the lonely. I hope she had no knowledge of our putting tubes down her throat and tugging at her clothes. We did what we thought was best, but did it help her to die with dignity and in peace? She would probably have said 'Oh, you doctors and nurses are so wonderful'. Could we have explained why that might not be so?

In the afternoon I have a problem presented to me by one of my doctor colleagues. He calls me into his room and says he'd like to tell me about a case. I like this colleague, Michael, a lot; he is thoughtful and considerate and doesn't bawl me out on his bad days.

He has seen a patient who is new to the practice. The patient is a young man who is a community worker. He is an asthmatic and had come to renew his regular prescription for inhalers. Michael asked if he smokes and was informed of a 30-a-day habit. Michael suggested that were he to give up smoking he might not need his inhalers. At this point they both became angry. The young man insisted it was his right to have prescriptions and to smoke. Michael thought it was his 'right' to refuse to give prescriptions.

Should I have been angry, asks Michael, or was it unreasonable? The incident clearly worries him a lot, reflecting his concern to be reasonable to patients. I do not have a simple answer, but we talk about the consultation and I can, at least, tell him that I would probably have felt the same way that he did.

Thursday

Two visits are in our day-book for me today. I don't often do visits, seeing most people in the surgery, but I have been asked to do 'routine follow-up' in these two cases.

The first visit is to an elderly lady to check on how she is and whether she is taking her tablets. She has high blood pressure and is being treated for it. Noone has told me anything about this lady other than her medical history.

The place is difficult to find. It is number 4a, a ground floor flat. A hundred cats (it seems) suddenly appear as I knock on the door. It is opened by the woman's daughter, whom I recognise from the health centre. Apparently she lives with her mother.

The smell of cats is overwhelming. It is warm outside, but the flat is even warmer. It is dark and dirty. In the midst of a seemingly chaotic mixture of newspapers, cats' litter boxes and half-empty packets of food, sits a bright and cheerful elderly lady eating what could only be described as a heart attack on a plate (chips, eggs, bacon and sausage, in fat).

A cigarette box and matches lie beside her. Her daughter resumes her seat by the blazing gas fire and finishes lunch while we chat. Yes, the pills suit her fine when she remembers to take them. No problems with housekeeping or eating — her daughter looks after all of that. I feel slightly queasy from a combination of fat, smell and heat.

I wonder whether there's much point in checking her blood pressure or indeed whether that is going to do her any good. I make some tentative enquiries about her diet, which turns out to consist mostly of chips and comforting chocolates.

I consider the pros and cons of talking about the link between diet, weight, high blood pressure and heart disease. She is in her seventies so in fact her long-term prognosis will not be altered substantially by such advice. Should I tell the daughter? My own middle-class, high-fibre lifestyle makes me unable to appreciate the joys of this dark and smelly environment with its fattening diet. Yet, undoubtedly this pair are quite content. Should I intervene? Will I add anything to the quality of their lives? With all the indecision I can muster I defer any action to the next visit.

My next visit stuns me. It is a 30-year-old single woman who, two years ago, set fire to herself in a housing office in protest against their failure to rehouse her. She survived, but her face, I had been told, was badly scarred. The doctor, who referred her to me, said she was depressed intermittently and didn't cope well with life.

Nothing prepared me for the devastated face I saw. The scars are numerous and disfigure her face. Her nose has been almost completely destroyed, she has only one ear left, eyelids have been remade and there is a lipless hole where her mouth should be. I say I have come to see her, to talk over anything she wants to, and to help in any way I can. Seldom have I been aware of what meaningless phrases I was using, as I was then. How could I help? What on earth would she like to talk over?

Her name is Susan. She lives, unhappily, with her parents. At the moment she takes a sleeping pill five times a day to take the edge off her consciousness, and also an antidepressant. She doesn't want to live anymore, she says. Life is over for her. She has no children and no boyfriend — how will she ever find a boyfriend now?

Nursing is, I believe, an art and science developed to assist people to cope with disease (of any sort) with which they cannot cope alone. But I feel I have nothing to offer Susan in coping skills. How can she learn to cope with her appearance and her lost future?

She shows me a picture of herself as she used to be — an attractive young woman. I ask her about her parents, relatives, friends, and religion. She seems to have so little in the way of affection and love.

After an hour I say to her that I would like to come to see her again, even though I don't think there is anything I can do for her. She says yes, come again. I go back to the clinic feeling inadequate and unimaginative, and talk over my visit to Susan with the doctor who usually visits her. He tackles the problem with enthusiasm from a medical perspective — maybe we should change her drugs, or we could refer her back for more cosmetic surgery more quickly than is planned. All of this is useful; but is it the care that will benefit Susan most? It seems to me that what Susan needs more than anything is to be loved and valued for the person she is, even with her profound disfigurement. Yet that is my view, not hers. Could she ever be helped in a way that would give her some positive feedback about her appearance? I get the impression that my doctor colleague actually feels as helpless as I do and maybe that is why he asked me to visit her.

Friday

Some 'regulars' come in today. Jean is 35, once married but now living with a known criminal (burglary) and alcoholic. She is an alcoholic and used to use other drugs.

Eight years ago her children were taken into care and subsequently adopted because she 'wasn't a fit mother'. Jean mourns for her children, sending them birthday and Christmas presents and trying to see them — a policy discouraged by Social Services.

I used to get the impression that Jean came in to see me, and at the same time was drunk and abusive to the receptionists, because she had nowhere else to go. Her man treated her badly on the whole, though he often came with her if she was injured (usually by burns, knife wounds or through being beaten). I had a soft spot for Jean, and was always glad to see her, however dishevelled she was.

All changed last year. Jean became pregnant and was ecstatic. She gave up drink, soft drugs and almost stopped smoking. She had a happy, healthy little girl called Rosa, on whom she dotes. Now it is Jean and Rosa who come to see me. Today Jean is angry with the hospital — Rosa hadn't put on enough weight and the paediatricians were concerned that she was failing to thrive. With Jean's previous history of being an 'unfit mother', she is labelled for life. I am not surprised that she lost her temper with the consultant, thus probably jeopardising her chances further. We talk about what the paediatrician has said and what it might mean. Rosa is there and I weigh her and give her a quick examination. She is lively and cheerful and doesn't look like an abused child at all. I tell Jean that and reassure her, I hope. Perhaps I identify too much with her: I would be as wild as she if someone suggested taking my children away from me. I phone her probation officer with her permission, and tell him Jean is concerned. I think it will be OK for her.

Another regular visitor to my room is Margaret — a large expatriate Irish woman. She came to lose weight in the first place, but now I think she comes because she can talk about her problems. She certainly isn't losing any weight. I always try to dicover *why* people over-eat. With Margaret, questioning released a storm of resentment about her life. Her husband is West Indian and goes out a lot, leaving her lonely. She has a daughter who left home but is now back with Margaret and her two children.

Today Margaret seems depressed. I say this to her and she starts to cry. It seems that this week she discovered that her daughter is a heroin addict, on a large dose of the drug. The daughter, on being discovered, left her mother's home and has disappeared. Her two children, who went with her, have now been taken into care.

Margaret's daughter is not the daughter of Margaret's present husband, so now Margaret feels alone and helpless. 'I wish she were dead,' says Margaret,

'I hope the police come and tell me that soon.' I try to focus on the children — where are they? Can Margaret see them?

Today Margaret is negative and uncaring. I hope next week she will be coping better and I ask her to come back sooner if she needs to talk to someone.

The third regular visitor is Daphne, who has for many years worked on a boring factory assembly line, in appalling conditions, for low wages. She first came to see me because she wanted to stay off work. She then kept coming back for the same reason — different minor complaints, but all necessitating time off work. Eventually I asked her if, in fact, she might be better changing jobs if she felt so loath to go to work. She agreed, but said what she really wanted to do was to be a nurse. We talked over ways in which she might do that, and I haven't seen her since. Today she comes in brightly, smiling — an uncharacteristic demeanour for Daphne. It transpires that she has got a weekend job as a care assistant with the elderly. The pay is bad but she loves the work, and can't wait to get to work now.

She wants to make it a full-time job but as yet there is no vacancy. She will hang on until there is. 'Thank you, thank you, nurse, for everything' she says, and I tell her it was really her that cured her own 'disease'. In fact, that's usually the case — people sometimes need help to identify the enormous resources and potential that they have within themselves.

Is this what nursing is all about?

Changing Ideas in Health Care
Edited by D. Seedhouse and A. Cribb
© 1989 John Wiley & Sons Ltd

Chapter Thirteen
Teaching Communication Skills to Medical Students

DAVID METCALFE
Department of General Practice
University of Manchester
UK

> When a person who is ill, or believes himself to be ill, talks to a doctor whom he knows and trusts, in the intimacy of his own home or the consulting room, that is a consultation, and it is the basis of medical practice.

> (Sir James Spence)

Introduction

Consultations are often perceived as relatively simple and straightforward transactions between persons who have clearly defined roles and whose relationship is tightly prescribed by custom and convention. Information is the stuff of the interaction. Facts are elicited by history-taking and examination for the purpose of diagnosis. The nature of the diagnosis and the proposed treatment are then communicated to the patient. This stereotype seems to underly conventional medical education. But the stereotype is a travesty of reality! It is not an exaggeration to claim that the doctor who can consult well has survived his or her medical education and then, nearly always, learned for him- or herself.

The mismatch between the way doctors are taught and the job they find themselves doing can result in the adoption of coping strategies. There appear to be high levels of certainty in the university courses, and yet doctors are faced with low levels of certainty in real practice. This is highlighted by the difference between the experience of treating relatively passive teaching-hospital in-patients and encounters with autonomous people attending health centres or out-patient departments. Where coping strategies are adopted to restore or regain control of a disconcertingly ill-defined and indeterminate situation, the effect on patients can be compounded by added authoritarianism and directiveness. Since conventional medical education is dominated by hospital-based specialists, few of whom have questioned the reality of the stereotype, there is little scope for change.

The Consultation — How Can Students be Equipped for Reality?

Byrne and Long, Pendleton, and Heath, have shown by rigorous research that a consultation is a complex interaction. Not only does it go through various phases, but both participants have their own agendas, which may overlap but are unlikely completely to coincide. There is also a frequent need to retrace steps, and there are mandates to be negotiated and permissions to be given, in a subtle interplay of tacit exploration. Both parties are trying to resolve tensions, implicit in the situation, between the role they would like to be playing and the actuality they face.

Underlying this interplay are two serious imbalances that might reasonably be expected to make any transaction between two people difficult. These are (i) that very different levels of arousal are experienced by the doctor and the patient, and (ii) that vastly different amounts of power are possessed. For a doctor to consult without recognising these complexities is to risk failure, not only in building a trusting relationship with the patient but in the central task of diagnosis and treatment. For a medical school to turn out graduates without an understanding of these central features of the consultation is a betrayal of the students' and the public's trust that medical students will be taught to practise good medicine.

The imbalance in arousal

The imbalance in arousal is, to a varying degree, inevitable. What is for the patient usually a matter of anxiety — what may be wrong? How serious might it be? What will I have to go through? — is for the doctor a routine task. Indeed, it is in some ways important for the doctor to maintain a degree of detachment while trying to make a coherent pattern out of the symptoms. Naturally these symptoms are described and given emphasis in terms that reflect the patient's feelings about them as much as their timing, intensity, and associations. But the patient's interpretation of, and feelings about, the phenomena presented are as important as the symptoms themselves. Not least because those feelings need to be given due weight. They also need to be reinterpreted to the patient when negotiating agreement as to the nature of the illness. Finding out about such interpretations and feelings requires sensitivity, and the development of empathy. The process is valued by the patient as evidence that the doctor is interested in him or her as a person. Estimable as these virtues are, the importance of bridging the arousal gap is not purely to do with the relationship, but also contributes to the efficiency of the consultation. This is because it allows for the exchange of clearer data. Of even more importance is the fact that exercise of empathy and sensitivity forces the involvement of the doctor as a person. There is a degree of self-exposure, and the doctor risks being hurt or rejected, and risks having to share pain or terror. The cool professionalism of detachment and objectivity, albeit presented with courtesy and sympathy, that is said to be the desired outcome of traditional medical education ('You must never become emotionally involved with your patients') rules out the creation of an acceptable balance of arousal.

The imbalance of power

The other major imbalance is of power. The doctor is, by definition, of social class I: 92 per cent of his or her patients are from social classes II, III, IV and V. The doctor is expert: patients are inexpert. The doctor must appear to be healthy: the patient will usually appear to be poorly. The doctor is usually on his or her own territory: the patient is usually away from home. A majority of doctors are male, yet women have higher consulting rates.

High social class, specialist expertise, health, and being on your own territory and maleness are all power factors. The imbalance is usually reinforced by the physical accessories of the consultation: relative positions, chair type and height, and territory all tend to reinforce the doctor's power. Once the patient is undressed, exposed, and lying down, the imbalance is further accentuated. In what other interaction, apart from another very ancient one, can a professional say to a client 'all right, stop talking and take your clothes off'? Signalling that it is time for the patient to be examined, and signalling the end of the consultation, usually by withdrawing eye contact and starting to write a prescription or the order for a test, are moves only the doctor can make. This reveals an enormous power that, if misused, can sometimes be quite brutal.

A map of patient care

The doctor may have the power, and may be comfortably distanced from the patient's angst, but that is not to say that he or she is not stressed. Figure 1 presents a two-dimensional conceptual model of the tensions inherent in patient

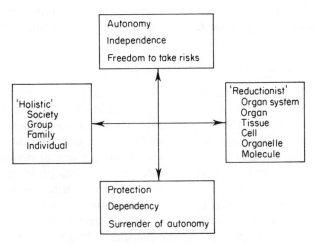

Figure 1 The tensions in patient care.

care. The horizontal axis represents the tension between 'disease centred' and 'patient centred' medicine, and the vertical axis, the tension between 'patient power' and 'doctor power'. The care of the patient in intensive care or the operating theatre can be positioned in the lower- right-hand corner. That of a person being rehabilitated after acute physical or mental illness will be placed mainly in the upper-left-hand corner.

The doctor is under continual stress, sometimes compounded by conflict with the patient, as to whether he or she is working in the right part of the 'map' or graph. Most of the time both doctor and patient are treading familiar ground, and what tension there is, on either axis is of the creative sort rather than stressful. However, where the situation is unclear, or the patient unwilling to conform to expectations, the doctor who has been trained in the conventional manner will probably respond to uncertainty by trying to take the transaction to the right and downward, not least because the upper-left area is *terra incognita*. While patients might be expected to be straining to get back into the top-left quadrant, and usually are, this is not always true: dependency and protection may be attractive roles. There is a common perception that if you are ill it is someone else's job to get you right.

Inappropriate expectations, for instance, of the efficacy of high technology care, may lead the patient to seek a disease-centred mode of care (Kubler and Ross's 'bargaining' phase in terminal illness). The likelihood of collusion between such patients and doctors who feel comfortable only in the bottom-right corner are clear. The risks of medicalising non-medical problems are considerable and expensive. Sometimes invasive, and therefore dangerous, tests are performed, inappropriate drugs prescribed and taken, and work on the real problem remains undone. Health care costs soar, particularly in those systems in which, unlike the NHS, there is direct access to specialists. To be able to move, sure-footedly, into the proper quadrant requires that the doctor has not only a wide range of skills, but also confidence in choosing which to use, and the ability to plan and change to a fall-back strategy should a skill not be effective. Flexibility is compromised by anxiety, and flexibility (which is evidence of humility) has never been seen as a goal of medical education!

Person-centred medicine and patient power

The concepts of person-centred medicine and patient power are relatively new. They owe their formulation within medicine almost entirely to general practice/ family medicine; and without, primarily to articulate patients and social scientists. These concepts are still, to some extent, unrecognised within what might be called the medical establishment. Whether or not people in the past were more prepared to be the passive, respectful, and grateful recipients of care, today's people, well resourced by the media with information and coming from a less instinctively deferential society, are not. As soon as the subject of medical care is recognised as a person, rather than a 'case', a container for disease, or a disordered organ, or 'the gall bladder in bed 10', then considerations other than those pertaining to pathophysiology come into play.

All people have basic personal and social needs, and health and illness have to be seen in that context, rather than as isolated phenomena. A succinct way to appreciate these needs was offered by Abraham Maslow (1970) who pointed out that people's ability to learn was related to their position on a 'hierarchy of need'. Put simply, if you do not know where your next meal is coming from, your energies must be directed towards survival, and not to Pythagoras or French irregular verbs! At the bottom of the hierarchy a person has no 'personal space'. As one rises through the hierarchy from survival to security to advancement up to full self-actualisation one has more space at every level. Space is essentially freedom, and in particular freedom of choice (what to wear, which show to go to, the books to read, the holidays to go on, the job to change to, the relationships to foster). It is also the capacity to grow, to reach one's potential. Perhaps 'space' is a useful working description of the idea central to the WHO definition of health as 'complete physical, social, and psychological wellbeing'. Feelings of personal space are intimately bound up with one's self-image: the more space you have the better you feel about yourself. This concept is essential to the practice and teaching of person-centred medicine. Not only can illness be seen to restrict or diminish a person's space, so that the maintenance or restoration of space becomes a legitimate objective of care in addition to the correction of pathophysiology, but some forms of care may themselves reduce the patient's space. This may be by reduction of autonomy, by the inculcation of anxiety to the extent that it limits the range of choice, or by direct effect on the body-image, itself an important component of the self-image. This is not to say that such space-reducing forms of care must be abjured: there may be no alternative if life is to be saved, or some quality in the life remaining preserved. But the loss of space inherent in the treatment must be considered and minimised. Respect for the patient's space is an ethical principle and is perhaps easier to understand than 'autonomy' (see editorial) *per se*. There is often a tacit or explicit mandate from the patient to surrender autonomy in the expectation of other benefits. Once the concept of space has been grasped, however, even patients in intensive care can be seen to have need of some, and will have given no mandate for its total removal.

The achievement of effective care with the minimum expenditure of resources depends on consulting skills that include lessening the arousal imbalance, some handing over of power, the recognition of the need to defend or increase the patient's space, and the ability to work in the right part of the 'map'. But how can these skills be taught?

Teaching consultation skills

Essentially skills are taught by a sequence of demonstration, supervised practice and feedback. This is how, for example, the elicitation of physical signs is always taught. Curiously, 'history taking', which is really a higher order skill, is seldom taught this way. Conventionally students are told what questions to ask, and go off alone to do it. They then present their findings (not always in the presence of the patient) and are judged by the extent to which the information they recount agrees with that held by the instructor! Every student remembers the chagrin experienced when there is a disagreement between the history he presents, which he is sure was what the patient told him, and the belief held by the instructor. The assumption is always that the student's story is the wrong one. Brief reflection suggests that this is actually unlikely for two reasons. First, the student's history is more recent (patients 'tune' the story each time they tell it), and second, there is good research evidence to suggest that patients feel most able to talk to the lowest member of the professional hierarchies with whom they have to interract.

Teaching history taking or the wider concept of consultation skills, should be carried out by the proven cycle of demonstration, supervised practice and feedback. Two practical facilities are of crucial importance: (i) closed circuit television and (ii) small group work. Whereas in the elicitation of physical signs the patient is inevitably passive, this cannot be so in the conversation that constitutes history taking. The presence of the instructor, a person of seniority and status, is certain to interfere with the transaction. With the patient's permission, a television camera can give the instructor supervisory capability without distorting the interaction. It also allows replay and analysis, which 'sitting in' doesn't. Small-group teaching has been shown to be an effective way of learning problem solving, and the best way of inculcating desired attitudes. Essentially, the students in a small group undertake a task together, and in achieving it learn from each other. It is the instructor's job, by choice of task and the way it is presented (by providing information on request and by modulating the discussion) to manage student learning, rather to teach didactically. As far as attitudes are concerned, the student can easily dismiss those recommended by the teacher by claiming that 'It's only a matter of opinion'. But the dynamics of a friendly and trusting group are such that he or she must eventually conform to the values of the rest. If the instructor finds at the end of a session that none of the group have come to espouse the attitudes he or she would have liked, the first task is to examine how secure those attitudes are, and if reassured, the discussion can be reopened on the next occasion.

The subjects of video-recorded consultations may be 'real' patients, simulated patients or other students playing the role of patients. All have been used, in one medical school or another, since the late sixties, and each has its fierce protagonists.

'Real' patients   'Real' patients fall into two categories: those attending for care on the day and who give their consent; and those, selected for the nature of their illness and their articulateness, who are brought back especially to 'help our young doctors to learn'. The former category has the advantage of total validity such that the student quickly forgets the recording camera. The disadvantage is that because the instructor cannot control the case mix, he or she has little control over the learning achieved — since the sort of case he or she wants to use to examine the skills involved is unlikely to turn up on the morning of the teaching session. There is also the risk of an ethical problem;

this might happen if the patient presents a problem with which the student cannot cope. For example, the student may have asked an open-ended question that has allowed the patient to open up about a major and distressing psychosexual difficulty. If this occurs the instructor would have to 'rescue' the consultation and take it over. This would force the patient either to extend to the instructor the mandate given, in good faith, to the student, or to withhold it from this new doctor arriving as it were from nowhere, thus compounding the pain of exposure with failure to gain help.

The real patient brought back for teaching purposes allows good control of the case mix, with little risk of anything going wrong. They may, though, become 'professionalised' in the way they respond to students, either by colluding (in the fashion of the old-time regular examination patients) or by making it hard for a student to whom they take a dislike. There is a fine balance between giving the patients sufficient briefing, and actually 'programming' them to the point at which they lose their validity.

'Artificial' patients   Simulated patients are of three sorts: actors (professional or amateur); members of the teaching staff; or (a sub-species found mostly in North America) people who have made a hobby or profession of simulating patients. The last group expect to be examined, even intimately, and are often trained to mimic the signs of specific illnesses, so they are often used for learning the skills of physical examination rather than the consultation as a whole.

The skill of the actor is essentially to 'become' the 'patient' to such an extent that he or she can be relied on to respond to the doctor as that person would. The advantages of using actors are that the learning case mix is controllable, that they know what the instructor wants to come up in the subsequent discussion, and that the 'patient' cannot get hurt. Knowing this the student can be bolder, relieved of the anxiety related to using a sick person to learn on. The disadvantage is that everyone concerned knows the patient is not 'real'. Although most students claim that they forget that the person before them was not a 'real' patient within seconds, when pressed in subsequent analysis of their style they can always say 'But I wouldn't have done that with a real patient'. It is vital that the instructor and the actors largely share the same assumptions about consulting skills and the underlying values: this necessitates plenty of preliminary discussion between them.

When members of the teaching staff play the patient, advantages accrue from their control of the case mix, and from the clues and challenges that they are able to offer to the student. The disadvantages come from the fact that students find it much harder to 'suspend disbelief', that the power imbalance is replicated, albeit in reverse, within and without the consultation, and that staff come from the same narrow social band that the students do, and therefore may find it difficult to achieve verisimilitude when playing a socially deprived patient.

The professionalism of trained simulators is different from actors: they are craftspeople rather than artists, and are mostly concerned to get all the features of the illness right. The advantages of control of the learning experience may be offset by this lack of validity. One would expect that, in situations where they expect to submit to invasive examination, their defence is the same as the patient: 'Its not me, just a piece of meat', which precludes the role identification that actors can achieve. Again there is a potential ethical difficulty because the student knows that the undressed and exposed patient is not really a patient and so is deprived of his or her emerging immunity to, or control of, sexual arousal.

The last category of 'patients' for these exercises is other students. There are many disadvantages: real embarrassment and shyness in youngsters without experience in the Thespian art may shade off into deliberate game playing: validity is minimal, and the students' own privacy could be put at risk if his or her briefing accidentally trespasses near sensitivity areas. It does, however, offer one advantage that none of the others do: the chance to savour what it is like to be a patient! For these reasons student role playing should be used only in concert with other methods.

Teaching through 'artificial' consultations   Before describing the way these facilities can best be used for teaching the skills and attitudes discussed above, it is important to make clear that this teaching method is perhaps the most difficult there is. The instructor has to review his or her objectives for the session, and work out from them the briefing, both of the student and of the 'patient'. He or she then has to watch the consultation as it unfolds, where necessary making notes of points to be injected into the discussion, while keeping an eye on the rest of the group if they are watching. Once the consultation is over the instructor has to run the discussion, keeping a balance between positive and negative feedback (that is, protecting students from being hurt by self-criticism as well as by that of their peers, while not losing the learning opportunity afforded by sensitively identifying errors). He or she must also ensure that each of the students gets a chance to contribute. Group dynamics have been described as 'listening for a gap into which you can insert your ideas for peer review'. All this must be done while mentally assessing the extent to which the objectives are being achieved!

Facility in teaching consultation skills is important for reasons that are not only educational, but also political. Traditionally, any innovation in medical education is fiercely challenged by the conservative members of staff, and student gossip about sessions that fail is joyfully accepted as ammunition. One of the characteristic paradoxes of this aspect of academia is that innovation is immediately challenged to prove its validity and effectiveness: something never required of the established and conservative disciplines, even if they have not been reviewed in ages!

The other general consideration is the way the 'patient' is employed after the consultation. This will to some extent depend on which type is involved. If it was a student he or she will be involved in the group discussion, as will a member of staff. It should be noted here that it is hopeless to try to act as the patient and the group tutor. But what about 'real' patients, and actors or 'simulators'? Some teachers do not allow 'real' patients into the group discussion, on the ground that they might 'hear more than was good for them';

others bring them in at the start but then, having given them their say, allow them to leave. Some teachers have them in throughout the discussion as active members of the group, whether still in role, or as general 'lay advocates'. Extrusion of 'real' patients may be justified to some extent in terms of avoiding their 'professionalisation' and thereby, if they are to be used frequently, losing validity. But actors and 'simulators' grow quickly, if well used, from being rather sophisticated visual aids to being powerful teachers in their own right.

A practical difficulty   It is interesting to note how ingrained the students' learning assumptions are. Unless carefully and specifically briefed they see the exercise as a diagnostic puzzle: 'I wasn't fooled by all the psychosocial stuff, it was obviously thyrotoxicosis' or 'In real life it would obviously be a straightforward diagnosis of gout but here of course I knew you'd put in some psychosocial problem'! Medicine has become for many of them a sort of intellectual game in which the prizes go to the one who 'gets' the diagnosis, regardless of the logic employed, regardless of how the patient has been treated, or how acceptable and practicable the management proposed. Their value systems, in many cases, have been changed by the way they have been taught. Briefings for these exercises therefore must make clear that what is under review is their ability to create a good working relationship with the patient, because that is a necessary skill not only in the making of diagnoses (because it will enhance the quality of the most important information available for that purpose), but also for planning management sensitively enough to obtain 'compliance'.

Because these learning methods are most often deployed by the 'soft' disciplines such as psychiatry and general practice, it is important to establish the pertinence of what is learned through them to all the other clinical disciplines. For this reason it is strategically wise to build each role on, or use real patients with clear-cut physical illnesses, while focusing the teaching on the impact of the disease on the patient and the amount of space that can be restored to him or her.

It is interesting to examine this concept of 'hardness' and 'softness' for a moment. As students see it, the hard disciplines provide them with proven factual material that can be presented to examiners, whereas the soft disciplines seem to be conceptual, vague and arguable. The traditional didacticism of 'the great white chief' inhibits their critical faculties, even though much of clinical medicine is unproven. Even when their teachers pass on the clinical wisdom 'There's no always and no never in medicine' they are betrayed by the inanity of the multiple-choice question! But if the 'hard/soft' concept is viewed from a more general standpoint it can be seen that 'hardness' is a prerequisite of the longest established disciplines that have not only the greatest political power within the school, but the strongest examination sanctions.

Balance   The Venn diagram (Figure 2) is a useful *aide-mémoire* for the instructor taking a consultation skills workshop, whether with real or simulated patients. By ensuring that some discussion takes place in each of the Venn circles he or she can maintain balance and, more importantly, provide the

This diagram indicates the four basic areas of activity in the consultation:

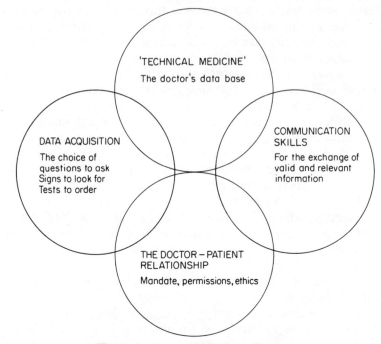

'TECHNICAL MEDICINE'
The doctor's data base

DATA ACQUISITION

The choice of
questions to ask
Signs to look for
Tests to order

COMMUNICATION
SKILLS

For the exchange of
valid and relevant
information

THE DOCTOR – PATIENT
RELATIONSHIP

Mandate, permissions, ethics

Figure 2 The teaching Venn diagram.

students with an understanding of the way these activities interrelate. This should prevent them thinking that only the technical medicine and data acquisition are important: indeed it should be seen that work in all four areas should be indissolubly woven together! It is unlikely that it will be possible to get good discussion in each area in every consultation reviewed, but it is the instructor's task to make sure that in the session some work is done in each.

The balance in activity will depend on where on the 'learning curve' the student starts. Where there is early didactic teaching about the psychology of the consultation, and instruction on such topics as the importance of eye contact and the use of open-ended questions, it is noticed that far less energy needs to be invested in the communication skills circle *per se*. Where such things are new to the students it is in that circle that a lot of time has to be spent, at least in the early stages.

Given entry fairly high on the curve, learning takes place on two broad fronts: hypothesis generation and testing ('technical medicine' and data acquisition); and the patient as a person (communication skills and doctor–patient relationship). Starting prompts for the first front include 'What are the possibilities?', 'What do you need to know to support that idea?', 'Why did you ask that?' The other students in the group can be encouraged to offer hypotheses, and to improve the database by asking their own questions of the patient (if included in the group) or simulator (while still in role). On the second front the prompts are 'tell us about this patient as a person', 'give us a thumbnail sketch of the patient's life', 'what did the patient want to know, and how did he or she signal it?', 'did the doctor negotiate to extend his or her mandate?', 'was the patient told the truth?'. Interestingly the amount of time students are prepared to invest in the doctor–patient relationship circle, if they find the group valuable, suggests that they have appreciated the opportunity, unlikely to have been afforded elsewhere, to discuss things that they feel are important. Indeed, the intensity of such needs when they surface can make it very difficult for the instructor to maintain the broad-front, four-circle balance, but that remains an important goal.

Concluding Remarks

Not only does this sort of teaching fill in gaps in the students' learning that should not be the sole responsibility of the departments most likely to be providing it, but it may actually challenge what they have been, or will be, taught elsewhere. Ideas such as defending the patient's autonomy, enhancing their personal space, sharing power and telling the whole truth, may be seen as anything from Quixotic to anathema by the more deeply conservative clinical teachers. The sort of teaching described here, with its emphasis on the importance of empathy, flatly contradicts the often spoken advice 'Don't get emotionally involved with your patients'. Of course, in a medico-legal sense this is quite right, but extended to mean 'Don't let yourself care' it is destructive. Of course it is difficult to bear the load of suffering and frustration, and a young doctor must find ways of coping with this if he or she is to remain effective, but to tell him or her not to care is to invite maladaptation by choosing to be detached, cool, and controlling. This presents the instructor with the delicate task of teaching the students while at the same time protecting them from retribution if they try to use what they have learned in a unit that is less patient-centred. This is rather like planting seeds that you do not want to germinate until the weather is warmer! A useful example is the issue of physical contact for comfort and communication: the held hand, the arm round the shoulder, the shoulder to weep on, or the cuddle. A lot of doctors quite often use these very human responses (it is important that they are spontaneous rather than calculated, instinctive rather than intellectualised), or find themselves crying with a patient. Many doctors agree that it was several years after they graduated before they felt secure enough to 'let themselves be human'. They find that it gives them a sense of freedom, and they feel that their patients value their humanity enormously without ever taking advantage of their vulnerability. Nevertheless, such behaviour is seen as most undesirable by some clinical teachers, who are likely to reprimand, sometimes quite destructively, students they find trying to comfort a distressed patient. (A recent paper (Firla, 1986) on student stress found that a third of the class were significantly stressed, and that the most common stressor identified was the way they were treated by consultants!) They would regard the process of teaching students to allow themselves to respond to their own emotions as downright subversive.

The strategy to correct the extensively reported shortfall in doctors' clinical behaviour, both technical and interpersonal, must be radically to redesign the medical school curriculum and the way it is taught. We are the products of our education and training. It has been argued that the problem starts with whom we let into medical school in the first place, and this may be so, but the large majority of those who we do admit are, at the outset, idealistic, sensitive and inquisitive: excellent material to work with. But fundamental curricular change seems almost impossible, so entrenched and powerful are the defenders of the status quo, and so inimical to change is the method of resourcing. Money, staff, space and equipment are distributed in some sort of equivalence to curricular time/student numbers; but they are used as much as possible to pursue the research on which the department's status and its members' promotion prospects rest. It is not surprising that no one gives away curricular time!

Recommendations

Within the conventional framework the tactical effort should go to more widespread and better resourced use of consultation skills teaching. This should have as its objectives that the student on completion should be able to:

1. Respond to patients' presenting symptoms, logically acquiring data to test each possibility.
2. Negotiate an effective, acceptable and practicable management plan with the patient.
3. Discuss the situation with the patient in terms that allow the patient to accept the situation and make appropriate decisions.
4. Work within the mandate he or she is given to enhance the patient's space and preserve the patient's autonomy.

Surely this is an adequate description of good medicine.

References

Byrne, P.S. and Long, B.L. *Doctors Talking to Patients*, HMSO, London.
Firla, J. (1986) 'Levels and Causes of Stress in Medical Students'. *British Medical Journal*, **292**, 1177.
Heath, C. Personal communication.
Kublen Ross, A. *Of Death and Dying*.
Maslow, A. (1970) *Motivation and Personality*. Harper and Row, New York.
Pendleton, D., Schofield, P., Tate, P. and Havelock, P.B. (1984) *The Consultation: An Approach to Learning*. Oxford University Press, Oxford.

Index